Train LIKE A MOTHER

Other Books by

Dimity McDowell and **Sarah Bowen Shea**

Run Like a Mother: How to Get Moving—
and Not Lose Your Family, Job, or Sanity

Train LIKE A MOTHER

How to Get Across Any Finish Line—
and Not Lose Your Family, Job, or Sanity

by Dimity McDowell and Sarah Bowen Shea

Andrews McMeel
Publishing, LLC
Kansas City • Sydney • London

Andrews McMeel Publishing, LLC
an Andrews McMeel Universal company
1130 Walnut Street, Kansas City, Missouri 64106

www.andrewsmcmeel.com

ISBN: 978-1-4494-0986-9

Library of Congress Control Number: 2011932649

12 13 14 15 16 RR2 10 9 8 7 6 5 4 3 2 1

ATTENTION: SCHOOLS AND BUSINESSES
Andrews McMeel books are available at quantity discounts with bulk purchase for educational, business, or sales promotional use. For information, please e-mail the Andrews McMeel Publishing Special Sales Department: specialsales@amuniversal.com

To all the other
mother runners out there

CONTENTS

INTRODUCTION

While we were Running Like Mothers, Sarah and I talked on the phone. Almost daily; 75 percent of the time we talked about work; 25 percent of the time, we didn't. And we wrote about a gazillion e-mails.[1] As we divvied up Facebook responsibilities, thought up new T-shirt slogans, and pored over flight schedules so we'd arrive around the same time to a race city, we had a cloud hanging over our heads. Namely, what book to do next. The prevailing thought we had was a running log, where you could write your mileage and daily victories, and we could entertain and inspire you with short essays and advice.

There were a few issues with a log, though. First of all, neither one of us has ever really used one. Hard to get behind something you're not sold on yourself. Secondly, in case you haven't noticed, the world is dominated by iPhones and laptops (and NikePlus and dailymile and the like) and other gizmos that have basically replaced the pencil and paper. Hard to get behind something you're not even sure will sell.

A face-to-face conversation at the 2010 Nike Women's Marathon, the place where *Run Like a Mother* all began 3 years prior, got some creative juices flowing. We thought of having little icons/spots to notate your period, your family members' birthdays, and your runiversary (the date on which you started running). While we laughed at the idea of a little line drawing of a tampon, the question still hung over our head like a thundercloud: Would our community of badass mother runners—one of the best tee slogans we came up with, by the way—use a log?

Then, during an event at See Jane Run in San Francisco, we asked a great group of women if they'd use a log. Despite one sweetly saying, "I'd read anything you two write," the overall response wasn't overwhelmingly encouraging. Still, we put together a proposal, but we never got around to sending it to our agent.

---

[1]Alas, none of them are funny or interesting enough to include here, as we did in the introduction of *Run Like a Mother*. Kind of like how your e-mails to your husband, before he was your husband, are all funny and creative, after you tie the knot, the messages get distilled: "Pick up eggs on the way home, please." Or "Megan is coming over for dinner." Or "Unclog the toilet today."

Around the start of 2011, the log felt as heavy as a real log. That we were carrying on our shoulders. During a 6-mile run. So I called SBS, and we had a conversation that went something like this:

Dimity: "We have to do a real book, Sarah. Even though we both get a little nauseated thinking about the amount of work it'll take to get it done, there really isn't another option. A log isn't going to fly."

Sarah: "You're right. [Long sigh.] I've just been avoiding saying it out loud."

And like that, our RLAM Training Log, which we'd been swishing around for about 6 months, got spit out like a long-run loogie.

As the log loogie fell by the wayside, *Train Like a Mother*—the other book we'd been talking about—started lacing up her shoes. Like a runner staring down her fourth 15-plus-mile marathon training run, we were reluctant to get the party started because we knew exactly what was ahead of us: a feeling of trepidation and dread as we figured out our route; doing the same motion over and over; the need to create our own "fun" as we ventured into areas we'd covered plenty of times; a work cycle that starts out with joy, turns into a grind, and then, once the finish line is near, feels both exhausting and exhilarating.

But, like that runner, we knew we had it in us to get it done, and we realized we were fortunate to be able to craft, in cinematic speak, a sequel. When we wrote *Run Like a Mother*, we invited you into our little house of running, told you not to mind the mess of our lives, and asked you to stay awhile. You did, and as you hung out, you told us stories, which we love and never tire of hearing. Tales of strung-out, stressed-out women reclaiming themselves through rhythmic steps on the pavement; of survivors who have triumphed over cancer, rape, divorce, abuse, and many other life speed bumps, thanks to the strength and power they gained through running; of moms suffering from postpartum depression who use their miles as a tool to reaffirm their purpose in life and sense of self; of friends who met by chance and, through countless runs together, are now the closest of sole sisters; of mother runners who have tested their self-perceived limits by taking on 2 miles without a walk break, a 5K in under 30 minutes, a half-marathon for the first time.

Although the stories are as varied as the running outfits we wear, they share a common, powerful theme: Running transforms us into happier, more confident, more patient, and, yes, badass women. (Or, as Elle Woods, the heroine of *Legally Blonde*, says, "Exercise gives you endorphins. Endorphins make you happy. Happy people just don't shoot their husbands; they just don't!")

As you took off your shoes and sipped from your water bottles, you asked questions about this running thing that had become—or always was—an integral part of your life. No question was too basic, too personal, too off topic, or too much information. "What is a split?" "I cut my 14-mile run short by 2 miles, and now I'm really bummed with myself. Should I go do two more right now?" "I'd rather spend my money on running clothes than everyday clothes. Is that weird?" "I've been sick for five days—thanks, preschool germs!—and missed my long run plus two others. Should I repeat my training week or just continue on?" "I want a training plan that isn't beginner but isn't going to kick my ass. Ideas?" "Why do I need to pee as soon as I start running when I already peed *right before* I left my house?"

And that is why, despite the dillydallying we engaged in a year ago, we committed to writing *Train Like a Mother.* We've tried our best to hit every training- and racing-related question we (and you) could think of, but, as our kids tell us, we often make mistakes. Fortunately, we're still at the ready to answer questions. Join our Facebook page at Run Like a Mother: The Book; check out our website www.anothermotherrunner.com, an entertaining encyclopedia of all things running related; follow us on Twitter: @Dimityontherun and @SBSontherun; and find our Another Mother Runner podcast on iTunes. You can also e-mail us at runmother@gmail.com. Especially if you have an idea for our next book.

—Dimity + Sarah

01

RACING FOR OUR LIVES: **PART I**

By Dimity

I have half a mile left in this morning's run. For an experienced runner like me—I've been loping around for 20 years—a teeny-weeny, itsy-bitsy half of a mile is nothing, right?

Wrong.

Because this half a mile is actually 800 meters, or two times around a track I crash at a local middle school. I'm in the middle of a workout we runners like to call speedwork: a run, usually broken up into short intervals and recovery periods, that emphasizes pushing the pace. For me, the emphasis is on the latter half of the word. I grunt out 95 percent work to squeeze out a roughly 5 percent temporary improvement in speed.

I don't do speed well, either mentally or physically. I'm almost 6 feet 4 inches tall, and it would seem like my long legs, which sport a 36-inch inseam, should be an attribute: fewer steps and less effort to cover the same distance. Wrong. In reality, big, overreaching strides (or at least my style of lopsided, not very efficient, overreaching strides) promote injury, which I've learned the hard way too many times. Plus, my legs are *heavy*: I think each one of them weighs at least as much as my 5-year-old son, who clocks in at a neat and hefty 65 pounds. To add insult to potential injury, my head is as good at convincing my body to hang in that leg- and lung-incinerating red zone as my two kids are about eating hamburger–spinach casserole without gagging. Not good at all.

Still, I've already completed four 800-meter repeats—or 2 whole miles of speedwork—with a lap of an "easy" jog in between. Within 30 steps of the first 800, my arms tingled and my throat went dry. I resigned myself into accepting the workout on the third curve of the track, or about .375 miles through, before trying to channel a gazelle on the last straightaway. (Yes, I'm a bit of a math nerd when I run: Converting distances myriad ways gets me through the workout.) As soon as I hit the exact spot where I started, I stop immediately and collapse my hands onto my knees, a move I repeat after every 800. When I feel like I no longer need CPR, I begin my interpretation of an easy jog: walk at a mall-like pace for at least half a lap, then do a geriatric shuffle for the rest before pulling up, checking the time, maybe blowing my nose, finding a new song on my iPod, grabbing a swig of water, and otherwise procrastinating as long as I can.

On the second interval, in the hopes of turning an 800 into a 795, I hug the inside of the track so closely my left foot grazes the infield grass a few times.

The middle interval(s) of speedwork, or the third one today, are always the hardest for me to get through. By this point, I'm intimately familiar with how long and how hard each 800 feels (too long and too hard, if you're wondering). Plus, my legs are no longer fresh, and I haven't crossed over the imaginary hump where I can tell myself this is next-to-last or the last one. In other words, the workout is not coasting along a virtual downhill yet. "Just go," I tell myself when even I'm sick of my lollygagging. So I do, and count my way—10 steps on my right foot, 10 steps on my left—through the second lap. When I assume the stooped-over position after the third, which may or may not be a few steps short of my exact starting point, my legs start doing the Elvis shake. The vibrations are slowly convincing the rest of my body this speedwork stuff is bunk.

You might be asking yourself, as I do with almost every pseudo-speedyish step I take, "Why am I doing this? Why in the name of all that is good in the world am I, a mediocre, unnatural runner, out here at 6:13 on a Thursday morning forcing myself to lap a middle-school track—a place, it should be noted, that as a teenager I hated more than parties with those awkward Spin the Bottle kissy games?"

Good question.

Despite being a mediocre, unnatural runner, I am definitely a runner. I've clomped through two marathons (and have, despite pushing myself around the track, promised my so-not-interested-in-26.2-miles body that it will never have to endure another one), plenty of half-marathons, a variety pack of triathlons, and the occasional 5K, 10K, mud run, and relay. So I've lived a good running life. For most races, I'm content with following a basic training plan, which means workouts are two words long, like "6 miles" or "4 miles." There are no adjectives (fast, easy, tempo); no extraneous terms (strides, repeats, recovery); no terrain requirements (track, hills). I train with just one goal in mind: to stop running whenever the finish line happens to appear under my feet.

This, it should be noted, is an absolutely fine way to train. The likelihood of getting injured is fairly low, and motivation to get out the door is conversely high. Heading out and knowing I can run 4 miles at the pace that feels right today feels quite lovely and simple. If I know, however, I have 4 miles of hill repeats—or worse, 4 miles of speedwork, during which I stare at my Garmin more closely than I watched my kids around a pool when they were toddlers—then I obsess about the workout. I dwell on it as I brush my teeth the night before. When I get up to soothe my son after a monster dream in the middle of the night, the number of repeats echoes in my head. In the morning, I try to talk myself out of it. As I approach the track, I get a little throw-up in my mouth. On most days, speedwork feels worse to me than getting a cavity filled and my brows waxed at the same time (something I have never done, by the way).

That said, I have randomly cranked up the training intensity for a handful of specific races during my running career. There wasn't any definite, common trend as to why I decided to go all hardcore on those specific events, with one exception: All of my tee-it-up races came after I had both of my children.

As you probably know, you have a kid, and everything that was once easy and a given, like a last-minute movie on a Friday night, a stretch of five whole quiet minutes between the hours of 3 P.M. and 8 P.M., or a shower after a run, is far from it. Although the challenges of motherhood provide plenty of opportunities to fulfill my daily need for feelings of accomplishment and pride—Look! I got one kid to soccer practice, one kid to karate, stopped at Walgreens to pick up a prescription, made it back to see one kid bow to his sensei and the other score a goal, and, well, it's quesadillas for dinner, but at least they're on whole-wheat tortillas!—the minute-by-minute maternal victories are simply not enough. Even when we do have a dinner during which the this-is-so-gross gags are limited to fewer than two per child, it's not like I walk away from the table feeling all victorious. More like, I'm just grateful I didn't have to deal with full-on drama.

On the other hand, running makes me feel like a rock star; when I return home after a few miles with a soaked sports bra and weary legs, I have the confidence, energy, rush, and ego I imagine comes with fans screaming your name. *Dimity! Dimity! You are so awesome!* More than 90 percent of the time, I am fine setting my run, mind, and body on cruise control and relishing the fact that 4 moderate miles provides me-time, an endorphin rush, and a chance to recalibrate my the-world-sucks meter back to neutral.

Sometimes, though, those basic miles land me in a rut, not onstage with Bruce Springsteen. When that happens, my motivation to get out the door is slim to none; if I manage to drag myself out, the endless miles seem to get incrementally slower. When I start feeling bitter about "seasonal" flags like hearts on Valentine's Day or tulips for springtime on the homes in our suburban neighborhood, I know I need a change. Last week, as I ran by a Snoopy flag, I had one of those

David Byrne–ian moments—you know, as in "This is not my beautiful life." *I drive a minivan. I clip coupons for Costco. I think new white tees from the Gap are a splurge. Ten P.M. is a late night for me. I obsess over my son's behavior in kindergarten. The last time I wore makeup was three weeks ago. What happened to the hip, make-it-happen girl I used to be? And why is she wearing Danskos now?* Two days ago, I was near the end of my run, when my endorphins should've been soaring up, not down. I should've been, "Rock on! This is my life! I love it!" when I saw Snoopy's ears flapping as he danced for Halloween. Instead, I wanted to rip the flag in half.

So today I am at the track in the hopes of nailing a 10K in 8 weeks.

I need a challenge to mix things up—to remind myself I am powerful and can create my own victories. Not only am I feeling blah about life in general, I'm also knocking on the door of Ms. 4-freakin'-0, and my metaphorical running life feels uphill now. As a sports and fitness writer for magazines, I've done enough stories on aging and exercise to know the latter slows the former at a near miraculous pace, but exercise isn't a miracle. Despite knowing how much work it'll take to get me to squeeze out a few drops of speed from these injury-prone legs, I'm resigned to my fate. I want—and need—a 10K hurrah.

Lest you get all freaked out and think this training thing is not for you, a beginning/not-serious/ superslow/not-talented/fill in self-deprecating adjective here (_____) runner, I, a not-serious/not-talented runner, am here to tell you it can be. Training can come in a variety of flavors—and I guarantee you never have to step foot on a track if you swore off them around the time you got your braces removed. Chances are, if you've run a 5K, you've already trained. At its root, training is about setting a concrete goal: namely, seeing the finish line and then pushing, persuading, and sometimes forcing yourself to get there. (Certainly you can train without racing, but IMHO it's kind of like cake without frosting: Where's the fun in that?)

Training means you head out the door with a specific workout in mind, whether it's 3 easy miles, five 800s, or a 20-miler to get ready for your upcoming marathon. Training means every run has a purpose: slower miles to build a cardiovascular base; hill repeats to increase leg and lung strength; tempo runs to enable you to run faster for longer; speedwork to fire up those fast-twitch muscles. Training hones your mind to handle discomfort, pride, dejection, boredom, and elation, sometimes all within nanoseconds of one another. Training means you might suffer more than you're used to. Training delivers all the benefits a regular run can—a slice of your sanity back; muscular legs that mean business; time with yourself, with girlfriends, or with Ira Glass; a sense of confidence and glee unmatched by other activities—but it ups the commitment level just a tad.

If training sounds onerous, I'll be honest: It can be, especially when I'm in the middle weeks of a training plan and the race seems light-years away. I wonder what's wrong with a few meandering miles here and there, missing a day or three of a weekly schedule, not being so freakishly driven. Then I remind myself the rewards of being on a plan more than make up for it. Training makes the splits on a Garmin drop faster than an almost-4-year-old drops her afternoon naps. Training transforms a pace that used to feel unbelievably hard into your new I-can-chat pace. Training gives you quantitative measurements of your improvement, when the rest of your life is blurry and difficult to pinpoint with any kind of progress. Training lets you feel a mini victory every day. But more than anything, training is a reminder that hard work gets rewarded. And you are worth the investment of time and energy. And the reward.

Running is a little like parenthood: The individual days and runs can be so long I wonder how I'll ever make it to 5 P.M., which is when I typically twist the spout of my currently hip boxed wine. But the years are a blur, going by so quickly I'm not even certain I can connect Point A with Point B. How can Ben, who it seems only yesterday took his first wobbly steps, be Velcroing his own shoes for his first day of kindergarten? Or how can Amelia, who I'm certain just learned to ride a two-wheeler, be suddenly doing flip turns in swim meets? Where did those days in between go?

Similarly, when I rewind through my running career, I'd be hard-pressed to remember a single workout more than a week old. I can't remember the training days or even many races. The highlights—the ones I visualize when I think of my running—are the races I really focused on and trained for. In a 5K in Denver, I remember the last leg-torching mile, with every cell of mine yelling at me to walk, but me telling the cells to, metaphorically, shut the front door. I was beaming when I called Grant, my husband, to tell him my time. I remember an Olympic triathlon: While the 10K run portion wasn't super impressive, I remember Grant, stationed near the 6-mile mark, telling me everybody around me looked like serious triathletes—and that I did, too. I remember, on my way to knocking almost 9 minutes off a 10-miler I had done the previous year, running down a hill as The Black Eyed Peas were telling me they "gotta feeling." I had a feeling, too: I felt like I was flying. My feet couldn't keep up with my body. I have goose bumps as I'm typing, and that race was 3 years ago. I remember a half-marathon 6 months after that where I blitzed my time goal and landed (for the first time ever) in the top third in my age group. In the 2 weeks following the race, I must have checked those results at least 20 times, just to, you know, make sure they hadn't changed.

That half-marathon? That was the last race I truly pushed myself in. It's time. After willing myself through the fourth 800, I uncork the last one. Within steps, my virtual gas warning light goes on:

My legs are hollering, my lower back is gradually tightening like a vise, my head is firing up a headache that will only gain intensity once the workout is over. I try not to think of any of it. I round one curve, which seems to have lengthened since the last interval. I battle the wind, which conveniently just blew in, on the first straightaway, and when I hit the second one with the wind at my back, I remind myself to hold something back: I still have one more lap to go. (This is a hypothetical statement. I've got nothing to hold back.) I hit the second lap, and I have only one 400—a single, measly lap!—of this heinous workout left. I fight the gusts and tell myself to just get to the second curve, where I'll take it home. The last stretch, I tell myself to "Go! Go! Go!"—which doesn't prompt an increase in speed but generally protects against too much of a decrease. I finish, toss out an f-bomb just to put an exclamation point on my effort, and, as usual, skip jogging a recovery lap. I have worked hard enough, thank you very much.

Instead, I take plenty of time gathering my goods. I walk (very) slowly to the parking lot, climb into my minivan, toss my water bottle onto the floor, which is littered with granola bar wrappers, pennies, crayons, and overdue library books, and head home to my little slice of suburbia, flags and all.

Satisfied with myself and my life, I am ready to start another day.

TAKE IT *From* A MOTHER
WHEN DID YOU FEEL LIKE YOU WERE A REAL RUNNER?

"When new ladies ask me a running question."

—KAREN (Not afraid to admit she likes passing people.)

"When I reached the 5-mile distance, after a year of never running past 3 miles. After that, I just knew I could push myself beyond my comfort zone."

—BETH (Loves her own treadmill: "I can run in a sports bra and shorts and belt out Lady Gaga.")

"Good question. . . . I'm still trying to figure that out."

—BRANDY (Began a walk-to-run program 10 months ago, and now logs 15 to 30 miles per week preparing for her first half-marathon. FYI, Brandy: In our minds, that's as real as a runner gets.)

"I thought I did when I lost my first toenail, but I really felt like a real runner when I ran an 11-mile training run solo with no music."

—CARYN (Proudest running moment: blowing her first snot rocket.)

"While running my first 5-mile race, a woman pulled up beside me and said, 'I've been trying to keep up with you for the past mile.'"

—CHANDRA (Trains on two-track farm roads that cut across wheat fields.)

"I think of other women as 'real runners' as soon as they start to run, but I didn't feel like a 'real runner' until I had been running consistently for a year."

—CHRISTY (Started running so she could order a bacon cheeseburger from Friendly's. "I was sick of staying within my calorie limit to maintain my weight, so I bought a treadmill for Christmas. My $5 cheeseburger ended up costing $705, but I am now a runner, and that is priceless.")

"I still don't think of myself as one. I'm just a mom who is trying to keep my sanity."

—JULIE (Has run 15 to 20 miles per week for the past 11 years, always on Tuesdays, Thursdays, and Saturdays.)

"I always have."

—KATIE (Started running alongside her dad when she was 8 years old.)

RACING FOR OUR LIVES: **PART II**
By **Sarah**

Despite my propensity to define myself by my race times, I don't always love to train. In fact, when I start a training plan, I resist like a horse that doesn't want to be saddled. The reins of the dictated workouts seem too tight; the burden of nailing certain speeds and times is too heavy. But within a few uncomfortable days, I'm tamed, and I love the certainty each workout brings. I know if I do what is laid out before me—run 5 miles; run 8 miles with the middle four faster; rest—I'll arrive at the starting line prepped and ready to deliver my best effort, which is what racing is all about for me.

I like a training run with a challenge, with extra speed built in or hills that need to be conquered. When I mentally flip through my toughest race-prep workouts, I get all nostalgic about them, like I do when I look through the velvet-lined box in which I keep my three children's lost baby teeth. There's the fog-enshrouded tempo run I did to get ready for the 2010 Big Sur International Marathon. The closer I ran to Portland's Willamette River on the 20-minute warm-up, the foggier it got. The river was invisible from the road overlooking it as I headed north to crank out 4 miles at a tempo pace around 8-minute miles. Damp, pine-scented air filled my heaving lungs as I recovered for 5 minutes before undertaking four more of the same speedy miles. In my mind, conquering 8 miles at 8:00 (or better) pace felt like an Olympic-caliber workout, something Deena Kastor or Kara Goucher would do. (Obviously the fog was clouding my perception of reality.)

Weather rules my memories, as another one that randomly pops into my head is a set of six 1-minute hill repeats I ran in the pouring rain for the 2010 Portland Marathon. As I pumped my knees and arms, trying to stay on my toes as I powered up a long hill near our house, I took note of where fat worms squirmed on the slick pavement. Retracing my steps on the decline, I briefly stopped to save the stranded buggers. I felt victorious on the way up, and noble on the way down.

Then there are countless track sessions for a variety of races that blend into one because I almost always ran them in the dark, long before the high school students started cutting across the track lanes en route to homeroom. My iPod was my sole companion as I looped the track once (400 meters), twice (800 meters), thrice (1,200 meters), and even four (1 mile) times, trying to maintain the pace of my fastest 5K race. I often told myself I could bail after four or five 800s instead of six, but my determination—plus Pitbull, David Guetta, and Cee Lo Green—usually kept me going. And I always felt badass when I dragged my weary butt home, steam rising off my lululemon capris.

My sports ego thrives on the paces nailed, the hills conquered, the laps completed. Thankfully, my (aging) body responds equally well. But I wasn't sure it was going to snap back after having kids: During the first run after the cesarean delivery of my boy–girl twins six years ago, I couldn't decide which hurt more: my still-healing C-section incision or my jiggling, milk-filled breasts. I was sure running would never feel natural again, and I'd never return to my pre-twins pace.

Instead, I've gotten faster. (Woot!) I've set all my racing personal records (PRs) since then because I focused on building speed as surely as I worked on getting tan as a teenager. (Hello, Peter Gabriel double-album cover lined with tinfoil to reflect every burning ray; hello, Johnson's Baby Oil.) Two years after fully recovering from the twin pregnancy, not to mention *mothering* two babies plus an older daughter, I got serious about training. I built up speed, and I honed it at the track, on the road, on hills, and in my head. My previous fastest mile time became, through about a year of focused work, the per-mile pace I could sustain over the course of a 10K race. No matter what was going on in the rest of my life—article deadlines for the *New York Times,* board meetings for the local twins club, or toddler temper tantrums times two—I knew I was in charge and, more important, I was improving.

Then comes race day, as unknown and unpredictable as a 4-year-old's birthday party. Will there be smiles or tears? Elation or disappointment? A sugar high or a meltdown?

A typical race morning usually starts out looking like a scene from a zombie movie: individuals or pairs of people walking down a deserted street, all headed in the same direction. I walk among them. I follow the crowd's lead, not exchanging many words but casting plenty of glances. As we draw closer to the starting area, I can hear an announcer telling people where the Porta-Potties are and how many minutes are left until the start time, then thanking the local sponsors. Inevitably, regardless of the weather, U2's "Beautiful Day" streams out of loudspeakers.

The race becomes real for me as soon as I see the starting line and its accompanying overhang, usually an inflatable arch or a draped banner. My nerves strum as I stake my place in the starting corral, sizing up my competition. That woman in the flowered black skirt looks like she did way more hill repeats than I did, and that guy over there reminds me of an older, balding Ryan Hall. I calm the butterflies by fiddling with my iPod, making sure I have the shuffle feature turned off. (I. Like. My. Songs. Played. In. The. Order. I. Set. Them.) Getting my Garmin GPS to lock in a satellite signal makes the final few minutes pass. A few quick pump-me-up jumps, the gun goes off, and the mass of racers starts moving forward.

I harness my enthusiasm, because I know I'll flame out if I let it carry me away. The song "The Lucky Ones" often leads my playlist, and Brendan James reassures me with his refrain, "We're taking a chance / We're the lucky ones / This moment is yours / This moment is mine / And we're gonna be fine." Of course I'll be fine, thanks to my training, but it's nice to be reminded. I wait for the more peppy songs on my playlist, which I position to start about halfway through the race, when I shift into fifth gear. Until then, a strong fourth gear is my aim. But like a five-page birth plan, an overly contemplated race plan can get dashed in an instant. Hotter-than-predicted temperatures can deplete my energy; a pre-race restaurant dinner can wreak havoc with intestines; the reality of elevation gains kicks in. ("So *this* is what 300 feet of climbing over a half-mile feels like, eh?") The pace that felt so comfortable at the beginning now feels as sustainable as cutting out all sugar from my family's diet.

My mind sees the holes in my training, not the whole program. Instead of envisioning the mile repeats I ran on my neighborhood streets, I regret the strides I often skipped at the end of easy runs. I chastise myself for not being diligent enough about hitting race pace for the final miles of long weekend runs. Maybe I should have rested instead of crosstraining every Friday. I definitely should have committed to that 7:30 P.M. Yoga for Runners class instead of hanging with the family after dinner.

With a small portion of the race left, in a semi-desperate move, I try repeating, mantra-like, "Just 10 times around the track; just 10 times around the track." But instead of motivating me, it makes me wince. Ten, or any other double-digit number, is too big for my sugar-starved brain to swallow. Instead, I down an energy gel to get my body back in the game because, even in my depleted state, I know weeks and weeks of training has prepared me for this, the hardest part of the race: convincing my brain I've got this.

I'd never finished a race wearing a smile as massive as the one I wore in the 2010 Big Sur International Marathon. Dazzling California sun surrounded me, and I was shining with delight—and a dollop of relief. Around mile 15, I had hit a rough patch. The start seemed so far behind me, yet I still had many miles to cover. Even the views of foam-topped waves crashing into steep cliffs couldn't buoy my flagging spirit.

Yet being a veteran of five previous marathons, including a 3:52 personal best just a year before, and about a dozen half-marathons, I was savvy enough to know I could keep mentally limping along or I could turn the race around for myself. I'd prepared so well and followed my 14-week training plan so closely, the decision was clear. Only my mind was struggling, not my body.

So I kicked out the mental monkeys, telling them the pity party was over. Despite weak math skills, I knew I was cutting it close to making my goal time of under 4 hours. (As you may already know, I'm forever striving for sub-4:00.) After that psychological turnaround, though,

I never stopped believing I could do it. Over the rolling miles that followed, I let go on the downhills, pushed on the flats, and strove on the uphills. I merely glanced at the strawberry stop near mile 21. A riot of orange California poppies blooming on a beach at mile 25 barely registered on my radar. As other racers decreased their speed to a walk on the quarter-mile-long, kick-in-the-teeth hill near mile 25.5, I kept pouring it on. The race was my greatest physical challenge since having to push for 6.5 hours during the birth of my first baby—yes, that period is correct: *6.5 hours,* not 65 minutes— and almost as emotionally rewarding.

I missed my time goal by a mere 93 seconds, but I was ecstatic at my effort. This may be hard to believe coming from the competitive half of this writing duo, but I swear, I was over the moon. On a natural high for days, I hadn't wallowed in my usual post-race letdown. The "Oh, nuts, it's over" blues and the "I could have done better" regrets—those unwanted guests who usually arrive moments after I cross a finish line, then linger for days or weeks—didn't surface.

I didn't let them. Before I even boarded the plane to go home to Portland, Oregon, I was debating which marathon to do next. And I wasn't sure what I was looking forward to more: the race or the training.

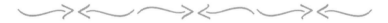

.1 SHOULD YOU RACE? **A QUIZ**
By **Dimity**

Not sure if you're ready to lay out a slice of your children's potential college fund just so you can pin on a race number? Here's a quiz to know if an entry fee is money well spent.

1 Your child(ren) is/are:

    A More than 3 years old.

    B Between 6 months and 3 years.

    C Under 6 months old.

    D More than one of the above.

2 Your motivation level these days calls to mind:

    A A rocket: always high, and I love to blast off! (And I'm so driven, I don't even notice how much my perkiness annoys other people!)

    B A minivan: steady and reliable, with a few visits to the shop for maintenance and unexpected breakdowns.

C A loose tooth: wobbly, and I can't find the courage to pull the trigger because I know it's going to hurt.

D I have to use a metaphor? What's that again? Anyway, I can't even remember how to spell the word—motivayshun?—let alone remember what it means.

3 The last time you fell asleep was:

A 10 minutes after putting the kid(s) to bed last night. Would've been sooner, but I needed to lay out my morning clothes and charge my Garmin.

B An hour after the kid(s) did last night, using those 60 minutes to check Facebook and scan newspaper headlines.

C Once waiting in the Starbucks drive-through and once with a baby attached to my teat. (I can't remember if those were two separate occasions.)

D After staying up to watch the Beijing Olympics closing ceremony.

4 You typically wake up:

A Naturally. My body craves its morning run.

B Begrudgingly after hitting snooze a few times.

C When someone screams.

D I'm pretty sure I've been half-awake for the past 6 years.

5 On an average day, how many familiar folks orbit into your personal sphere?

A Too many. With my job, school drop-off, and church group, I'm all talked out by the end of the day. Oh, and I teach a spin class and know everybody's name there, too.

B Fifteenish: I wake up next to my significant other; talk to at least two friends on the phone; go to lunch with three co-workers; chat up other parents at the playground.

C A handful: my neighbors, my mother-in-law, the cute, shaggy-haired Trader Joe's cashier. (Okay, I only pretend I know him.)

D One or two: my husband and/or my kid. Oh, make that three, because dogs are really just furry, four-legged people, right?

6 What did you eat yesterday?

  A Two pieces of toast with peanut butter; two packages of GU energy gel; protein flaxseed shake made with frozen cherries and bananas; an apple; two hard-boiled eggs; a Honey Stinger bar; chicken breast with brown rice and vegetables; steak and veggie fajitas, with guacamole, beans, and rice; and a large slice of peanut butter pie.

  B Two unadorned frozen waffles, post-run; the same leftovers for lunch and dinner: a great pasta dish with lots of veggie, all-organic goodness from Whole Foods; a peach; a handful of baby carrots; a 3 Musketeers bar. (Hey: I was at the grocery store solo . . . gotta take advantage, you know?)

  C A breakfast I can't remember; lunch was PB&J on slightly moldy bread (I just ripped off the green spots: It's all good.), a banana, a few fries from my kids' Happy Meals (we didn't have enough bread for them); and Raisin Bran and another banana for dinner.

  D Something between feeding my children, I'm pretty sure. And purse snacks of unknown origin.

7 Your last run was:

  A Two hours ago.

  B A couple of days ago. I went with a friend, and we did some fartleks just for fun. (Yep, that's my life now: fartlek = fun.)

  C I got in about half my 6-miler 5 days ago, but there was a meltdown in the stroller/daycare/ nap situation, and, well, I got in 3 miles, right?

  D Wait, what day is today again?

8 When is the last time you crossed a finish line?

  A Last week. And I'll cross one again in about two more.

  B Within the past 12 months.

  C After I had a child extracted from my loins.

  D Never. Or at least not in this century.

9   How intimidated are you to sign up for a race?

   A   Seriously? Next question.

   B   Not scared by the idea of a race, but a bit daunted by the self-inflicted pain that goes along with racing.

   C   I feel nauseated from the time I pin on my bib until I cross the starting line, but then I'm good.

   D   I'm petrified of coming in last. And not looking or feeling like a real runner.

10   The last goal you set for yourself was:

   A   Are you talking professional, financial, personal, family, or emotional?

   B   To read at least one book and to try four new recipes every month. So far I have a 3-month streak going.

   C   To get my linen closet organized before the end of the month.

   D   To make it to 5 P.M. before I crack open a beer. And I really don't like the taste of beer.

Tally your answers.

Mostly A's: Time for you to a) aim for a PR; b) take on a longer distance; or c) preferably both.

Mostly B's: Unsolicited advice: Give yourself the goal of doing a race longer than you think you can do. (We believe in you, and you should, too.)

Mostly C's: Get thee to a racecourse within the next 3 months, or risk experiencing the equivalent of an adult temper tantrum.

Mostly D's: Grab a friend, find a 5K, and do not pass go until you're standing at the starting line.

02

BEFORE YOU HOP ON THE TRAIN

By Dimity

I promise we won't retell too many stories we already shared in *Run Like a Mother*—remember that one time Sarah exercised for, like, 10 years straight?—but it's worth briefly recounting how this whole circus came to town. I was pregnant with Ben, our second child, and I knew a storm was brewing as my belly grew. My family has a history of depression, and as much as I tried to pretend I was a healthy, separate flower growing next to the diseased family tree, my genetic reality had come crashing down when I had Amelia, our first kid. Despite always wanting to be a mother, I couldn't embrace the role the way I pictured myself doing. On most days, I felt like a ghost hovering above my body, watching myself live my life instead of actually participating in it. I could socially engage for short playdates and grocery store greetings, but in actuality, all I wanted was a dark room, my bed, and endless hours by myself to shut my eyes and turn off my brain.

Because we had only one kid and because Grant, my husband, knew running was a huge factor in my well-being, not to mention the state of our marriage, it was relatively simple for me to continue running post-Amelia. (I didn't run through either pregnancy, and didn't fret it, either.) Although I denied it for most of my 20s, running has always been my antidepressant. When my legs are pleasantly exhausted and endorphins are floating through my body, I am able to see the world from a balanced perspective, not from 6 feet under. I rely on running for mental equilibrium to such a degree that my biggest concern isn't my splits or my mileage or my race schedule. It is the day that, for whatever reason, I won't be able to run anymore. I worry disproportionally about that impending news.

So I was pregnant with Ben, and Grant landed a job in Colorado Springs, which meant we were moving from our home in Santa Fe. We packed up our stuff and crossed the state line when Ben was 2 weeks old and Amelia was almost 3 years old—which meant no nearby friends, no daily companions but the kiddos, no idea where the grocery store was, no control over my swirling hormones and head, no place to go but down.

I plowed on, as I always do, but knew I was in a hole deeper than I'd ever seen before. I had an escape plan—I had asked Sarah about 9 months before to do a marathon—but flirting with a marathon via e-mail and actually committing to 26.2 miles are two different things. I can talk a good game, but I'm not always the best at taking action. Fortunately for me, things clicked into place, including an assignment for a blog and feature story about our training and race in *Runner's World*, which would become the seed of *Run Like a Mother*.

TAKE IT *From* A MOTHER
ON A SCALE OF 1 (NOT AT ALL) TO 10 (TOTALLY ANAL), HOW MUCH DO YOU PAY ATTENTION TO YOUR RUNNING FORM?

"I'd say a 6. My friend would say I'm an 8."

—ALISA (Dream running date: Jon Hamm. "I don't even know if he runs. I just want to hang out with him.")

"I'm slowly paying more attention to my form. I noticed the improvement in my form after my second 10K, when my dad mentioned my ponytail didn't swing like it used to. Now that's my gauge for whether I'm running well or not.

—CHRISTY (Repeats the words "power, energy, strength" when she does track repeats.)

"I'm a 6. I try to pay attention, but then I get distracted by a new song or some shiny object."

—COREY (Calls hills malevolent, cantankerous, power-sucking opponents, but loves them. "Give me a hill any day over a flat, boring stretch.")

"An 8. I often run with my shoulders up. I think it's from years of competitive swimming. To make them relax, I think about having sex."

—MELISSA (Eats hard candies on runs longer than 6 miles.)

"I'd say a 1, but I'm trying to pay more attention to it to see if it helps my knee problems."

—VICKY (Scared of the treadmill: "I've seen people on *The Biggest Loser* take those rolling falls off the end.")

I trained with Sarah virtually but knew I needed a real companion. I rounded up my soon-to-be-great friend Katherine, and we hit the roads. We started training in early May for the mid-October race; I wanted plenty of time for my far-from-primed body to ramp up slowly. Through lots of tears, unnerving thoughts, and frightening ambiguity about my life and my family, the marathon training was my life preserver. It kept me social; it kept me motivated; it kept me moving. So even when I got a stress fracture in my heel that kept me from running, I knew I had to keep going. I hopped on the bike in my basement and trained my guts out, pedaling with more vigor than I'd done anything in the previous 4 years.

It was a win–win situation. I emerged from the marathon with an amazing friendship and a sense of balance I hadn't felt in years, and the event launched *Run Like a Mother* and our business, Another Mother Runner. Although there's no way I would've believed it at mile 21, when I was positive the finish line wasn't worth 5.2 more miles of struggle, that race was, quite simply, the best thing I've ever done for myself.

As mom, wife, and freelancer, I spend my days doing things for other people. I write stories to send to an editor, go to the grocery store to feed my family, fold countless pairs of underwear for said family (not really true: I simply flatten and pile up the underwear), taxi to dentist appointments and the library to keep the kids' teeth and brains healthy. Just like I knew I wanted to be a mom, I also knew I wanted to be a wife and a self-employed writer, so it's not like I didn't sign up for this program. It's just that it's much more depleting than I ever anticipated it being. At the end of the day, I have nothing left to give; even laughing at Stephen Colbert feels taxing at times.

As I was reminded, once again, when I took on my second marathon, committing to a training plan is strangely liberating and energizing. Yes, I am adding to my "motherload," but I choose to put it on the list. What's more, I choose the race, the program, the places I'm going to run, the music I'm going to listen to, the shoes I'm going to wear. Nobody else gets to have input or place demands.

I choose this race for me. Repeat: *I* choose it for *me.*

That perspective is so different than wanting to please an editor, soothe a gaggle of children, engage a husband, ensure the dogs don't have heartworms. Instead of everybody else putting demands on your life, training forces you to stay within your own, individual box. Running on a regular basis makes you live in and appreciate your own body; fight your own physical and emotional demons; focus on your goal; and strengthen your resolve, your confidence, and, while you're at it, your muscles.

If it sounds like training is self-centered and narcissistic, it completely is. But if you're like 95 percent of the mothers out there, you deserve—and are in definite need of—some me time. And in

TAKE IT *From* A CARGO-PUSHING MOTHER: STROLLER STRATEGIES

When we heard that Dorothy, another mother runner, pushed a triple stroller for 13.1 miles, we contemplated building a shrine to her.

Here's how she recounts that epic run: "I told myself I would be happy with 5 or so miles that day. I wanted to beat the heat, so I woke up 3-year-old Miles, so he honestly was in a daze. He ate his breakfast in the stroller, then was pretty quiet most of the time. The baby, 9 months old, was asleep the entire time. Chloe, 5 years old, and I worked on math facts, including counting from 0 to 100. That kept both of us busy for about 5 miles. Then I pulled out a new trick: I asked her to tell me stories. She loves to talk, and she told me all sorts of princess stories. That bought me some more miles. Toward the end of the run, around mile 12, I said, 'Man, Mommy is tired!' Miles started cheering, 'Mommy, you can do it!' and Chloe joined in. They cheered me on the entire rest of the way until I hit 13.1."

In case you don't have kids—or legs—that are that happy for 13.1 miles, here are some tips from Sarah Johnson, a leader of Stroller Strides in Denver, and her posse of mother runners.

9 Your stroller should be the right height for you. The handle should come to hand height when your arms are bent 90 degrees, like you're running. If you're extra tall or petite, be sure the handle is adjustable or you'll sacrifice your form.

9 Speaking of form, even though you're pushing a load, your running form should be the same as if you weren't running: relaxed shoulders, not overly long stride, and extended spine and upright posture (avoid leaning from the hips). Keep your stroller close to you with slightly bent elbows, not at arm's distance away. Sarah recommends having a one-handed grip on the stroller, and alternating hands every minute or so. When you head up or down a hill, be sure to keep your toes facing forward and keep your footsteps quick and light at all times.

9 Keep yourself and your cargo safe: Use the safety strap at all times. Melissa, who is currently preggo and has a toddler, usually uses one hand, except for when she heads downhill. "Uphill, I like the challenge of one hand," she says. "Downhill, I like the security of two. That could all change, of course, when I push a double wide." (Hate to be the bearer of bad news, Melissa, but quite a bit more will change when you need a double stroller.)

♀ Give your kid a goal: Tell him you're going to run to the end of the path, until he watches one episode of *The Backyardigans*, or until you get to the park. That will limit, but sadly not eliminate, the "Are we there yet?" queries. (Even McDonald's can be the goal: One mother runner posted a picture on Facebook of her kids eating a Happy Meal as she ran. Obviously, you can't turn to Ronald for every run, but we applaud her resourcefulness.)

♀ Snacks! Save snack time for the stroller. A toddler's version of the slow-food movement is key. Fill up a cake ice cream cone with raisins and Goldfish, or GORP (good old raisins and peanuts). After she is done eating bit by tiny bit, she'll be able to chomp the cone. Licorice offers another good way to pass the time: Challenge your 4-year-old to practice tying a knot or pretending to lasso an imaginary horse.

♀ Entertainment! Just like the Happy Meal run attests, we condone doing what it takes to get it done. Some moms keep special toys allotted just for the stroller, so the child thinks being strapped in has its benefits. Others pull out their iPhones with kid-friendly apps and let their munchkins get all techy. Singing, playing I Spy, counting dogs, and looking at books are other ways to pass the miles.

♀ If you have a playground break planned, stop after at least two-thirds of your run is complete. That way, if they moan and groan on the way home, you're almost there—and you're assured of getting in most, if not all, of your workout.

case it all feels too greedy, consider this argument: If you are the linchpin of your family, you need to be healthy enough to fulfill your duties. You must take care of yourself, because, the sad truth is, nobody else is going to take care of you. Plus, if you're dragging and sad and bitter—which you might be if you're always last on your list—your emotional state will negatively affect your house and family.

With training come a couple of responsibilities, though. (Yes, I sound like a mother. That's because I am one.) First of all, there's the responsibility to tend to your body as you train. That means—try not to laugh—sleeping as much as you can, eating right, respecting your legs or lower back when they say that running might not be the best thing to do that day, and saying "no" to stuffing the weekly folders for your son's second-grade class because your schedule is already packed from before the sun rises to well after it sets. It's easy to hop on the train, focus only on the mileage, and Get. It. All. Done. At

Count YOUR STEPS LIKE THIS MOTHER
CLUE INTO CADENCE

Coming back from my second stress fracture, I knew something in my running style had to change so I wouldn't soon be feeling the agony of my third one. I bought the book *ChiRunning: A Revolutionary Approach to Effortless, Injury-Free Running*, by Danny and Katherine Dreyer, and studied it like I was cramming for the GRE.

Although the whole philosophy behind ChiRunning—super-engaged core, super-relaxed limbs, a slight lean forward from the ankles—is taking me longer to adopt than I wish it would, there's one component I immediately found helpful: paying attention to my cadence.

Cadence is the number of steps you take in a minute. You might have heard people talking about an ideal cadence of 90, which means each foot hits the ground 90 times in 1 minute. (This could also be called a cadence of 180; same diff.) If counting to almost 100 tires you out, you can figure out your cadence by counting the number of times one foot lands in 20 seconds, then multiplying that number by 3. If your right foot lands 25 times, for example, you've got a cadence of 75 (or 150); if it lands 27 times, your cadence is 81 (or 162). Experts advocate a cadence of 90, but I'll never get there; being tall and long limbed, 85 is my goal. I'm somewhere around 82 most days.

Why does cadence matter? Taking more steps per minute promotes smaller steps, which means your feet plant under your body, not in front of it. Every time you reach a leg out to land, your quad muscles contract and you're putting on your brakes, albeit ever so slightly. If you keep your strides short and plentiful, not only do you keep momentum on your side, but you land lighter on your feet, which helps keep injury at bay. People ahead of me used to turn around as I ran up on them when I was still four football fields away—I must have sounded like a T-rex—but now I sneak up on them. Well, not quite, but lately I've been met by more startled expressions, as if they hadn't heard my approach.

I actually own a metronome, a little device the Dreyers encourage runners to use that attaches to the waistband and can be programmed to beep on either every step, every other step, or, if I'm feeling waltzy, every third step. It's not exactly a pump-you-up beat, but the constant rhythm isn't as annoying as I expected. (It is, however, embarrassing when I pass another runner, so I try to turn it off. Now that I'm not *clomp-clomp-clomping*, I like to be completely stealth.) The beep, beep, beep actually pulls my head back inside my body, making me think about form. Strong arms, quick steps, relaxed legs, strong belly.

You don't have to geek out like I do, but next time you're feeling weary or achy on a run, figure out your cadence and incrementally work toward 90. That way, injuries have less of a chance of sneaking up on you. But watch out for me.

whatever junk-food, no-sleep, ignore-aches cost, because that's what we mothers tend to do. I've been there, done that, and will never go back again. While you can certainly do the same masochistic thing, I guarantee your finish-line experience, if you get there, will not be as self-affirming as it could be.

Second, there's a responsibility to your family. (Like I had to tell you that.) While you're feeling so good and striving and achieving, they—meaning both your significant other and your kids— might feel a little neglected, especially if your MO up to this point was making sure their worlds ran seamlessly. Keep the peace by sitting down with your husband and, if they're old enough to understand, your kids, and go over your training schedule. Again, I don't want to repeat too much from round one, so suffice it to say, it will be easier for everybody if you can keep the ripples your training makes to a minimum. That means getting up early, running while the kids are at school, taking your lunch break on the treadmill, or doing whatever else it takes so your training slides into your family members' schedules as effortlessly as possible. (I realize that's not the most women's lib–y thing to type, but life isn't always fair. I probably didn't need to tell you that, either.)

Finally, there's a responsibility to train responsibly. Running, like anything that makes you ultimately feel good, is addictive. The attraction is especially strong when you've broken through the typical beginner phases—not being able to regulate your breath, feeling ploddy during a run, and frustrated at the end of one—and are finally grooving. As a fellow addict, I'm definitely *not* telling you to run less or to compromise your running time, but I am gently suggesting you run and race intelligently. When I hear of people running monthly marathons or having similarly ambitious schedules, I get a little queasy: Not only do incessant 26.2s not give your body a chance to recover, but that schedule, by default, makes many weekends about you and your races. If you have a family that doesn't really get this running thing, this regimen can breed resentment. You likely have to travel, get to the expo to pick up your number, wake up early the following day, run for 4 or more hours, then spend the rest of the day recovering. That's not exactly a nice 5-miler before church, then brunch at your brother's house.

In my mind, it's better to be conservative with your races, instead of emptying your bucket as quickly as possible. Personally, I don't like to race a lot, so two half-marathons a year and maybe a

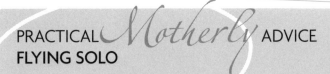

PRACTICAL *Motherly* ADVICE
FLYING SOLO

"I have mad respect for single moms, running or not," says Kelly, a mother runner who responded to a blog post we did about all the single ladies. "Mad respect. I don't know how you do it every day. I don't think I could."

Our sentiments exactly, Kelly.

Even though we occasionally get irked at our husbands when they hit Chick-fil-A three times when we're away on a business trip, the fact they are still in bed—and, theoretically, on call—when we head out into the darkness makes the drill that much simpler.

But whether you're a single mom, a military wife, or with a man married to his job, you can—and need to—get a run in. "I used to feel guilty for leaving my son at day care a little longer so I could run before or after work," wrote one military wife. "Now I know I have to take care of me in order to be able to care for him during the long months of deployment." Another mother runner echoed, "Running kept me sane through my divorce. The only way I could run was to go to the gym and put my daughter in child care. I accepted that running was just as integral to my happiness as spending quality time with my daughter."

Here are some preferred ways sisters are doing it for themselves:

STRATEGY 1: PAY FOR IT

⅋ The number one savior for all moms, single or not, is the treadmill. In addition to allowing you to get your run on when you're home and on mother duty, it's the no-out solution when outside is sporting bone-chilling or Sahara-like temps; when your only window to run is at o-dark-thirty (A.M. *or* P.M.) and safety is a concern; when you can't figure out how to squeeze in a run *and* watch *Glee*. Don't believe us? Take it from this mother runner's endorsement: "I *heart* my treadmill. Seriously. I can't imagine life without it. It keeps me sane; it gives me strength; it brings me peace."

⅋ Another option: gym child care. If you're about to join a gym, be sure you ask about child-care fees and hours before you sign on the dotted line. One mother runner wrote that she always maxes out the 2-hour limit, and has no guilt about it. "I live in a town where some people think leaving your kids for 2 hours is hazardous to their health," she preaches. "It is more hazardous to everyone for you not to get your mommy's-sweating time when you are doing everything else on your own." Amen.[1]

♀ Finally, let's not forget the babysitter. You can get in a quality run in an hour, which likely costs somewhere in the $10ish range (read: less than a manicure, a few trips to Starbucks, or a movie ticket). That money is some of the best cash you can spend.

STRATEGY 2: TRADE FOR IT

♀ If you don't have the funds for a babysitter or treadmill, that doesn't mean you're SOL. Barter for your run: Some mother runners trade hot meals with their child-free friends in exchange for babysitting; others ask older neighbors, who are familiar to all parties, to hang out when they run, then they help the seniors with snow removal or errands. ("Schedule it during naptime, and they can just read a book and drink coffee," advised one mother runner.) You may need to barter with the ankle biters, too. "I make my kids promise me that if they will give me 1 hour on the treadmill, I'll do what they want for the rest of the day," said one (more-patient-than-we-are) mother runner.

♀ Kid swap: You drop your kids off at your girlfriend's house, go get your sweat on, and as you stretch your hip flexors, she heads out. Or if your kids are grown, pay it forward. "My running partner has little ones, a job, and a firefighting husband," explained a mother runner of older kids. "I remember what it felt like to have a girlfriend offer to watch my babies so I could get outside and stay sane. I love being able to help her out now." Just use your help-me chips wisely. One mother, a military wife, runs only on the weekends that she's competing. "That way, I don't overuse my awesome friend who watches my son when I race," she explained.

STRATEGY 3: TAKE 'EM WITH YOU

♀ Although we wish, for self-serving reasons, that it was a woman instead of a man who came up with the idea of throwing bike wheels on a stroller, we still rank the running stroller as the second most important invention for running moms. (The sports bra is clearly first; the

---

[1] If you've got the funds, here's another option: "I found a young woman who really wanted to join the local club I belong to, so I paid for her membership. She stays in the pool with my two boys while I work out, then she can do what she wants," suggested the mother runner. "I have days I don't want to go, but I know she'll be there, so I get my rear out the door."

treadmill, third.) Strap those piglets in, take pacifiers, iPhone, fruit snacks, and anything else you'll need for soothing, entertaining, or eating, and remember that every mile you run is a good mile, simply because it's done.

9 Once the kids are either no longer complacent passengers or have become too *grande* to push, transfer them to a bike and do your best to keep up. A bike path is best to keep momentum at a maximum and disruption to a minimum.

9 Park your kids on the infield of a track (the long jump makes a good sandbox) or baseball diamond, and go round and round. "I had my kids predict how many laps I could do," said another mother runner. "The winner got a prize, plus their sweet encouragement helped me persevere." (No word on whether she threw the contest to have the kid who whined the least win.)

9 Use your village. "When my husband was traveling, I could sometimes convince my mother-in-law to spend the night so I could run in the morning," said one mother runner. Variation on the theme: You and the kids spend the night at their grandparents' house and you run while they're enjoying a pancake breakfast. Then everyone gets a sweet treat.

STRATEGY 4: GET CREATIVE

9 If you're cool with it, stash a baby monitor in your mailbox or next to the tree and run up and down your street. If your child is older, and you're lapping your street, tell him to come outside when he wakes up. Your offspring don't necessarily have to be asleep. "I did hill repeats up and down the block in front of the house while my kids took turns timing me," reported one mother runner.

9 Sneak it in: There's no reason why you have to be present at a playdate (unless, of course, you're the one hosting it); at a birthday party (2 hours at germ-laden Chuck E. Cheese's, when your kid doesn't even know you're there, is valuable running time); or at T-ball practice (games are a different story). You may inspire others to take back their time. "When I came back from my run during my daughter's dance class," wrote another mother runner, "there was a dad in the parking lot who had set up his bike trainer next to the open door of his minivan. He had a toddler inside watching a movie while they chatted and he pedaled away." Love that dad.

couple shorter races suits me well. Maybe you and your life can handle a marathon in the spring and the fall, or maybe you're all about staying short and local, so you do the 5K and 10K summer circuit and call it good. Or maybe you simply do the annual turkey trot with your kids by your side. You know your family and your body and both of their limits intimately by now. Without sacrificing what is important to you, do your best to keep them both balanced on the teeter-totter of your life.

Twenty years into running, I think I've finally got the balance thing down. I run three to four days a week: enough to mostly soothe my mind, but not so much that my body or family is pushed to the edge. What I don't have mastered is avoiding the emotional land mines that still can blast away at my psyche. We're done with having kids, so postpartum depression is in my rearview mirror, but I'm mature enough now to admit my blossom and my being are solidly attached to my greater family tree.

I'm not sure I'll ever know how to permanently level the roller coaster, turn off the tears when they spring for no reason, and cultivate the stability I so admire in others. However, I do know the best Band-Aid ever, and I'll keep putting it on until I can't do it any longer: I go for a run.

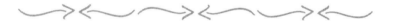

.1 THE LONG-LOST *BADASS MOTHER RUNNER HANDBOOK*
By Sarah

The other day, when I was cleaning out our minivan to get ready for a road trip, I found something I hadn't seen in years—the *Badass Mother Runner Handbook*, wedged under the middle row of seats. Its blue leather cover was coated with dried, sticky puddles of apple juice. When I cracked open the pages, pretzel crumbs fell out along with a Twizzler being used as an ersatz bookmark. The distinct odor of armpit emanated from it. This precious tome must have gotten left in the Odyssey after the 2007 Hood to Coast Relay. I was overjoyed it turned up, just in time to share some excerpted highlights with you, badass reader.

SECTION 1: RULES GOVERNING PERSON PUSHING A RUNNING STROLLER
Article 5

Any mother runner (or female friend of said runner) who pushes a stroller while running can count her mileage as double. Example: 3 miles becomes 6; 5 miles counts as 10. If the cargo includes four legs and four arms, she can quadruple her mileage.

Article 6

If the route is particularly hilly or covered at a rate that qualifies as "speedwork," the mileage can be quadrupled, e.g., 3 miles equals 12 miles on NikePlus or in running log. If it's a double stroller, then 3 miles equals 24. (And who said you'd never cover 20 miles?)

Article 7

The male significant other of mother runner does not enjoy the same multiplying effect as his female companion, as he has testosterone in his system. Clearly an unfair advantage.

SECTION 2: RULES GOVERNING OCCUPANT OF A RUNNING STROLLER

Article 14

Any high-fructose corn syrup consumed by offspring while sitting in a jogging stroller passes through the child's body undigested. The same is true with artificial colors and preservatives.

Article 15

If run is conducted at speeds exceeding 4 miles per hour, the energy generated from running automatically converts all consumed artificial ingredients into whole grains and fresh vegetables.

Article 18

Any iPhone apps played or television episodes watched by child in running stroller do not rot the offspring's brain; the exposure to fresh air, nature, and one-on-one time with mother negates the corrupting effect of mindless media.

SECTION 5: RULES PERTAINING TO EARLY MORNING WORKOUTS

Article 3

When, after an early morning run, another mother runner utilizes any quiet moments before her family awakens to stretch or foam roll in lieu of an uninterrupted shower, the flexibility and injury-preventing benefits are multiplied by 3.

Article 15

If mother can complete entire workout; get herself showered (including removal of unwanted body hair) and dressed; make family lunches; find library books and homework; oversee children getting dressed with hair and teeth brushed; ensure entire family consumes breakfast that includes carbohydrate, protein, and fruit; witness children getting on school bus; kiss partner; commute; and be seated at desk before boss arrives on a regular basis, please fill out online form for admission to Badass Mother Runner ranks.

SECTION 7: APPLICATION GUIDELINES REGARDING TREADMILL USAGE

Article 1

Running a long run (exceeding 90 minutes) on a treadmill lets you attain Silver Level of Badass Mother Runner (BAMR) status.

Article 2

If treadmill run of an hour and a half or longer is done without the aid of iPod, the *Today* show, or Netflix'd episodes of *Heroes*, Gold Level status is reached.

Article 3

If said treadmill is in unfinished basement with low ceiling and no windows yet you can still hear your children bickering (and your significant other ignoring them) in the family room above you, Platinum Level is attained.

SECTION 9: APPLICATION GUIDELINES RELATING TO WEATHER CONDITIONS

Article 14

Icicles on eyelashes merit fast track to BAMR status.

Article 15

Eyelids frozen shut on run instantly makes you a BAMR.

SECTION 11: APPLICATION GUIDELINES PERTAINING TO RUNNING WHILE PREGNANT

Article 1

Continuing to run while pregnant, despite the speed at which burgeoning mother runs, confers Badass status.

Article 8

Running half-marathon pregnant elevates woman to Gold Level BAMR status.

Article 10

Running on day woman goes into labor also raises her to Gold status. If water breaks while running, mother attains Platinum.

03

THE 5K:
THE FIRST STEP(S)

By Sarah

Unless you count the mile at fourth-grade field day, my first running race was a corporate challenge 5K, done with a bunch of my rowdy co-workers at a regional sports magazine. Despite spending our days writing about sports and fitness, none of us had specifically trained for the race. If memory serves right—this was 22 years ago, so cut me a little slack—we found out about the Wednesday evening race on a Tuesday. The husband-and-wife owners of the magazine had gotten free entries as trade for an ad in the magazine, so we figured, "What the h-e-double-toothpicks." My compadres and I were all in our twenties and relatively fit. I was an avid gym goer, another editor was a tennis player, and there were a few soccer and ultimate Frisbee players in our ragtag crew. Plus, we heard talk of free beer at the finish line.

I shudder when I recall what I must have looked like as we clustered near the start line along San Francisco's Embarcadero. I wore a pair of orange-and-white-striped nylon shorts that were almost short enough to qualify as bun huggers. (They were vertically striped, though, so I had that going for me.) On top, I sported a men's large white cotton long-sleeve tee emblazoned with our magazine's title across the chest. But more horrifying than the shirt's bagginess or the shorts' TMI must have been the look on my face—and the feeling of dread in the pit of my stomach. I was immersed in a sea of runners bouncing up and down and flapping their arms to stay warm as the evening fog rolled across the bay. The two other editors, Sue and Chris, were talking about what pace they planned on running, while I had no clue about how to pace myself or if I'd even be able to cover the entire distance.

After some corporate suit's welcoming remarks (which sounded to nervous me like the garbled wah-wah-wah way adults talk in *Peanuts* cartoons), the starting gun sounded, and we were off. I don't remember much about the actual race, but I distinctly remember how I felt after I crossed the finish line: elated. I'd just run my first race! I'd run the entire way, and I hadn't come in last. A victory.

PRACTICAL *Motherly* ADVICE
LET'S START AT THE VERY BEGINNING

By Dimity

We always say the world would be a better place if there were more mother runners in it. But how does one go from driving on the road to running on the road? With your help, of course. Here are a few tips for helping an interested but not yet convinced friend to get her run on.

⚡ Realize that, just like getting married or having a baby, there is no optimal time to change a lifestyle. So when she asks about running, don't reply with a murky, "Oh, yeah, let's run together sometime." Instead, jump through the slightly ajar door. Call her—or sit down with her—and map out when you're going to walk/run together. Aim for 30-minute segments, three times a week, for a few weeks. Then show up.

⚡ If she is coming from a mostly sedentary lifestyle, encourage her to start with 3 weeks of walking, four times a week for 30 minutes. That's a good foundation to get her going on our 5K: Finish It plan (see page 33).

⚡ When it's time to run, have her go small. The 5K: Finish It plan starts with 2 minutes of running. If that feels like too much, 1 minute or 30 seconds is fine, too.

⚡ Have her go slowly, too. Running, to many nonrunners, hearkens back to a near-death intensity, à la the 100-meter dash way back in grade school. Lay out only one rule: When you run together, you have to go at a pace at which she can converse—or at least answer your questions with more than a "yes" or "no."

⚡ Remember, your runs together are about her, not you, so don't think of her miles as your workout. Instead, use the days you run with her as your easy, recovery days; get in a run before you head out with her; or ask her to join you for the final miles of one of your long runs. If you're marathon training, plan to meet her at mile 15 of your 18-miler: You'll love the company, and she'll get to see that everybody eventually slows down. Try not to freak her out by telling her stories about your riotous intestines or the swath of skin rubbed raw by your new sports bra.

9 When the going gets tough for her—and it will—remind her running is hard, and every athlete gets down on herself now and then. Carry a tiny velvet hammer: Be sympathetic, but also be sure she gets (most of) the workout done. She might hate you temporarily, but ultimately she'll love you for many miles to come.

My virgin race experience—including, um, not remembering a thing about the actual race—is not that unusual. The 5K is a perfect race for beginning runners, for gym rats who want to spend more time on the treadmill, for you to accompany a friend who needs a booster by her side, and for seasoned racers looking to add a speedy dash to their endurance training.

While I don't recommend jumping into a 5K with a single day's notice like I did at age 24, it *can* be done. Whether you're crossing your first or your 21st 5K finish line, the training doesn't eat up a ton of time, since the longest you'll need to trot is 30 minutes. Translation: Your family will barely notice you're missing before you walk back through the door.

Short training doesn't mean inconsequential training, though. The miles you put in for a 5K are plentiful enough to produce tangible changes, such as a looser waist in your jeans, better moods, and enhanced confidence. If you're a beginning runner taking on a 5K for the first time, you will likely see a smaller number on the scale. If you're gunning for a 5K PR, you will likely see a lower number on your Garmin. But as you reap the benefits, you won't lose ground in other places; your boss, whether a business school graduate or a preschooler, won't comment on you being tired, drag-assy, or nodding off at your desk.

Three point one miles is the perfect distance to taste success as a beginner—long enough to elicit pride as you cross the finish line, yet short enough to prevent flameout—as well as to push yourself if you're a more experienced runner. Paradoxically, a 5K race actually gets harder as you get stronger and faster. Instead of cruising along with a smile on your face as newbies do, you crank and crank with a scowl contorting your mug. Maybe this is why many runners move on to longer distances after a few 5Ks: a prolonged yet lower-intensity effort can be more comfortable than the short-but-extreme stints. Or maybe many intermediate and advanced runners move past the 5K, feeling it's an entry-level distance.

I encourage you to sideline that attitude: Just because you have crossed the line on some 13.1- or even 26.2-mile races, don't think you're beyond 3.1-mile ones. Pushing yourself hard, without letting your foot off the gas, for 5 kilometers is a challenging thrill. What's more, a 5K is also an excellent

TAKE IT *From* A MOTHER
ARE YOU AN INTROVERT OR EXTROVERT ON RACE DAY?

"I'm a total introvert. I don't want to chat. Smile and nod at me. That's all I want."

—COREY (Elected not to buy the race photo of herself retching on University of Colorado's Folsom Field.)

"I'm an introvert until the gun goes off,
and then I find myself gabbing with everyone."

—TERRI (Her second half-marathon, a tough course on which she had to take
walk breaks and got blisters, left her depressed for a while.)

"I talk sometimes, but usually just try to breathe. I did a race 6 weeks after
my first daughter was born and felt I needed to explain to everyone why
I was doughy, slow, and had leaking breasts. I chatted a lot that race."

—HEATHER (A minimalist on training runs: "I don't even carry water.")

"I listen to music, but I'm also an extrovert—possibly to the extent that others find
me obnoxious. What can I say? All my solo running catches up with me, and when
I'm in a race, I have to chat it up with other racers, the race officials, the fans."

—PHOEBE (Occasionally struggles with a sudden "need to go" during a run, so before a
race she normally takes a couple chewable Imodium tablets with lots of water.)

"Definitely an introvert. I'm in the zone, so don't bug me."

—MICHELLE (Keeps track of her race times: "It would drive me batty if I didn't.")

"I thank volunteers, and also yell out what kilometer
we've passed when I'm racing in the U.S."

—KIM (A Canuck who is working on silencing her inner voice that tells her she's too slow.)

"In life, I'm a total extrovert, but on race day, I'm mostly an
introvert. This is a mystery I'm still trying to figure out."

—TARA (Sex the night before a race? "Ha. Good one.")

tune-up race for almost every other distance; it builds the endurance of newbie 10Kers and hones the speed of half- or full marathoners.

Still need to be convinced? Even if you blitz through the course, the recovery from a 5K won't slow you down like a 13.1- or 26.2-mile race will. Those longer events can leave you hobbled, in that painfully good way, for days, and make you scale back your running for weeks, if not a month. Instead, after a 5K, you can down some chocolate milk, hop in the shower, and be good to go for a full day of family fun. Better yet, your kids might be able to do the race with you. Many 5Ks cater to families with fun runs for younger kids and courses that older kids can tackle. You run, they run, and then . . . ta-da . . . naptime for everyone in the afternoon. Talk about a win–win.

I promise, I'm not trying to shill a Snuggie, PajamaJeans, or other infomercial gem, but I'll be honest: After that inaugural effort, I didn't do another 5K race for nearly 20 years. I moved on to 10Ks, a half-marathon, and then focused on marathons, rowing, and, oh yeah, having kids. For whatever reason, I decided distance was more appealing, and I forgot the allure of shorter races.

Two decades after that 5K in San Francisco, I stepped back into the distance at the U.S. headquarters of Nike, not far from my Portland home. The race was a fund-raiser for local schools. (Another selling point of 5Ks: They often benefit charitable organizations, so you can help out a cause in a fun, pro*active* way.) Phoebe, my older daughter, was in kindergarten at the time, so she was set to run a 1-mile race after my 3.1-mile one. There was a party atmosphere at the start. I waved at some other parents I knew, then gave the thumbs-up to my fam on the sidelines.

Since I was, by then, a veteran of numerous other races, my stomach wasn't clenched in a fist as it had been in the City by the Bay. This time, in the lead-up to the race, I'd followed an 8-week training plan. I'd honed my speed somewhat, yet I didn't have much of a race plan. When I spied Kelly, a friend in a bright green tank top, I decided to keep her in my sights throughout the race. Or at least try to.

Within the first few steps of the race, I had an alien experience. I felt light on my feet. At 5 feet 11 inches and 163 pounds, it was a new sensation for me; I decided to go with it instead of question it. I veered to the outside to pass a group of runners, and I turned on the gas once I cleared them. Kelly, in kelly, was only a few steps ahead of me. Along a straightaway, she started to pull away, but as we rounded a curve, I could see her brown ponytail bobbing. At the 2-mile mark, I stepped up my pace again and started to close some ground between me and greenie. A mile later, my lungs and quads were straining, but not with the overwhelming heaviness that often fills my legs in longer races. I crossed the line in 23:33 (thanks, Athlinks.com, for storing my times!), good enough for a surprising third in my age group. It seemed (heck, *seems*) so unbelievable, yet it highlights another 5K attribute: These shorter races often have fewer participants, so you have more room to run your own race and possibly end up with some accolades.

Later that day, as my 2-year-old twins napped, I stopped staring at my age-group plaque long enough to scour the Internet for upcoming local 5Ks. Still riding the post-race buzz, I definitely wasn't going to wait until I was in the 60-to-65 age group to rip up a 5K again.

5K: FINISH IT[1]

"A 5K is a nice blend of distance and speed. Plus, if you go out too fast, you're not completely dead at the end."

—ALISA

Best for: A beginner looking to test the waters of this training/race thing.

Physical Prereq: A couple weeks of consistent 30-minute-or-more walks, three to four times a week. No running experience needed.

Plan Overview: This 10-week program builds incrementally, through walk/run combos, to a 30-minute straight run before the 5K. All walk/run workouts are 30 to 35 minutes, but if you can swing it, add 5 minutes of easy walking as a warm-up and cool-down to sandwich your main workout.

1 What it says:

What you do: Regardless of how you have to reschedule your week, do not miss this workout.

More details: Although this plan is slightly repetitive, each session is vital because it helps prepare your heart, lungs, and muscles for your sure-to-be-spectacular upcoming running feats. Kind of like how a womb prepares itself for a bambino to grow.

2 What it says: 5 x walk 4 min; run 2 min.

What you do: Warm up by walking for 5 minutes. Then, walk briskly for 4 minutes and run for 2 minutes, and repeat the cycle for a total of five times. Cool down for 5 minutes. Done!

More details: Walk segments are at a brisk, steady pace. Runs should be done at a slow, easy, and comfortable pace. No heavy breathing. Save that for elsewhere—and, yes, your husbands can thank us.

---

[1] This plan, as well as the other seven running plans in this book, were crafted by Christine Hinton, a badass mother ultra-runner, coach, and all-around cool chick. Her website is therunningcoach.com.

5K: Finish It

Quick Key:

= Bail if necessary.   = Bailing is not an option.   XT = Crosstrain

WEEKS	MONDAY	TUESDAY	WEDNESDAY	THURSDAY	FRIDAY	SATURDAY	SUNDAY
1	[1] 5 x walk 4 min.; run 2 min.[2]	XT[3]	5 x walk 4 min.; run 2 min.	XT, or rest[4]	[5] 5 x walk 4 min.; run 2 min.	5 x walk 4 min.; run 2 min.	Rest[6]
2	5 x walk 2 min.; run 4 min.	XT	5 x walk 2 min.; run 4 min.	XT, or rest	5 x walk 2 min.; run 4 min.	5 x walk 2 min.; run 4 min.	Rest
3	4 x walk 2 min.; run 6 min.	Fun workout[7]	4 x walk 2 min.; run 6 min.	XT, or rest	4 x walk 2 min.; run 6 min.	4 x walk 2 min.; run 6 min.	Rest
4	3 x walk 2 min.; run 8 min.	XT	3 x walk 2 min.; run 8 min.	XT, or rest	3 x walk 2 min.; run 8 min.	3 x walk 2 min.; run 8 min.	Rest
5	3 x walk 1 min.; run 9 min.	XT	3 x walk 1 min.; run 9 min.	XT, or rest	3 x walk 1 min.; run 9 min.	3 x walk 1 min.; run 9 min.	Rest
6	3 x walk 1 min.; run 10 min.	Fun workout	3 x walk 1 min.; run 10 min.	XT, or rest	3 x walk 1 min.; run 10 min.	3 x walk 1 min.; run 10 min.	Rest
7	2 x walk 2 min.; run 13 min.	Fun workout	2 x walk 2 min.; run 13 min.	XT, or rest	2 x walk 2 min.; run 13 min.	2 x walk 2 min.; run 13 min.	Rest
8	2 x walk 1 min.; run 14 min.	XT, or rest	2 x walk 1 min.; run 14 min.	XT, or rest	2 x walk 1 min.; run 14 min.	2 x walk 1 min.; run 14 min.	Rest
9	Run 20 min.; walk 1 min.; run 10 min.	Fun workout	Run 20 min.; walk 1 min.;run 10 min.	XT, or rest	Run 20 min.; walk 1 min.; run 10 min.	Run 20 min.; walk 1 min.; run 10 min.	Rest
10	Run 30 min.	XT, or rest	Run 30 min.	Run 30 min.	Rest	5K![8]	Pop the cork!

3 What it says: XT

What you do: Anything but run. Aim for 30 to 45 minutes at a moderate-to-harder effort level on the bike or elliptical, or in the pool. (See page 112 for other suggestions.)

More details: If you're so inclined, feel free to throw in a few short bursts of higher intensity during your workout.

4 What it says: XT, or rest

What you do: Take your pick. It's best to crosstrain if you haven't been up more than once the previous night.

More details: Try not to let yourself off the hook too many times. In addition to helping you see the finish line of the 5K, we're secretly trying to get you into the habit of making a workout a part of your daily routine. (We're sneaky like that.)

5 What it says:

What you do: If need be, skip it.

More details: In an ideal world, you'll be so stoked from seeing your near-daily improvement that you won't miss many workouts. In this world, first bail on your XT/rest days before you skip runs. If all else fails, bail on the marked runs, but do your best not to miss more than two walk/run sessions in a row.

6 What it says: Rest

What you do: Lock your kids in the basement, put your feet up, watch a little TLC. J/K, dude, J/K. But you do need one day of no prescribed workout at least once a week.

7 What it says: Fun workout

What you do: Flip to page 116, pick your poison, and let the good times roll.

8 What it says: 5K!

What you do: Soak up the experience as you hustle your buns toward the finish line.

More details: Take a lot of pics: As your first race, you'll want to look back at them fondly.

TAKE IT *From* A MOTHER
DO YOU HAVE SEX OR A DRINK THE NIGHT BEFORE A RACE?

"Before kids: both; after kids: neither. Who can stay up for that?"

—JUDY (Motivates herself by thinking about the other moms running at 6:30 A.M.)

"I may have a glass of wine depending on where we eat and who we are with. Sex? That depends on the wine consumption."

—JOANNA (May or may not buy race photos: "Depends on how skinny I look.")

"My husband refused the night before my 10-miler. He said I needed to 'save' my legs."

—CAROLINA (Dream running date: Jake Ryan from *Sixteen Candles*.)

"Sex, of course! I know I will be too sore for it after the race."

—BOBBI (Began running when she was deployed to Iraq: "I was coming out of a bad relationship, plus there was the stress of being in a combat zone. Running seemed like the best way to save my sanity.")

"Maybe alcohol. No sex. What if I got hurt?!"

—KRISTI (Not good at crosstraining—minus bedroom acrobatics: "I either want to run or rest my legs.")

"No alcohol, but it's a reward post-race. Sex depends on how much I am asking of my husband on the day of the race. If it is going to be a long day for him with the kids, definitely."

—YEIKO (Still wears her sports bras from eighth grade.)

"My husband doesn't even ask."

—MELANIE (Scared that the seams on her favorite eight-year-old black Brooks shorts, a must-have for marathons, are going to split.)

"Hell yeah, both."

—MICHELE (After the initial post-race desire to vomit has passed, welcomes a post-race margarita.)

5K: OWN IT

"In my last 5K, I ran negative splits and finished with a kick I didn't know I was capable of. I felt like a rock star, passing everyone who had run out of gas."

—ERICA

Best for: More experienced runners looking to bust out a new personal best at this short-but-intense distance.

Physical Prereq: Your idea of a comfortable long run is at least 5 miles, and you have an established base of 15 to 20 (or more) miles per week. A prior 5K and at least a familiarity with the burn of speedwork is a bonus, but not necessarily a requirement.

Plan Overview: This 10-week program hones your speed in a variety of ways, from strides to sustained tempo runs to six Thursday track workouts. The long runs top out at about 8 miles, ensuring you'll have more than enough in your tank to keep the accelerator pushed down the entire 3.1-mile racecourse.

5K: Own It

Quick Key:

= Bail if necessary.

= Bailing is not an option.

CD = Cooldown
E = Easy
LR = Long run
RP = Race pace (see page 105 to determine yours)

T = Tempo (see page 213 for definition)
WU = Warm-up
XT = Crosstrain

WEEK	MONDAY	TUESDAY	WEDNESDAY	THURSDAY	FRIDAY	SATURDAY	SUNDAY
1	E: 4 miles + 4 strides[1]	[2] E: 3 miles; or XT[3]	XT	[4] 1 mile WU; 4 x 400 at current 5K RP w/400 recovery; 1 mile CD[5]	E: 3 miles	LR: 5 miles[6]	Rest[7]
2	E: 4 miles	1 mile WU; T: 2 x 1 mile, .5-mile recovery; 1 mile CD[8]	XT	E: 3 miles; or XT	E: 3 miles	LR: 5 miles	Rest
3	Fun workout[9]	E: 3 miles; or XT	XT	1 mile WU; 6 x 400 at current 5K RP w/400 recovery; 1 mile CD	E: 3 miles	LR: 6 miles	Rest

5K: Own It *continued*

4	E: 4 miles	1 mile WU; T: 2 miles; 1 mile CD	XT	E: 3 miles; or XT	E: 3 miles	LR: 6 miles	Rest
5	E: 5 miles + 6 strides	E: 3–4 miles; or XT	XT	1 mile WU; 3 x 1000 at current 5K RP w/400 recovery; 1 mile CD	E: 3–4 miles	LR: 7 miles	Rest
6	E: 5 miles	1 mile WU; T: 3 x 1 mile, .25-mile recovery; 1 mile CD	XT	Fun workout	E: 3–4 miles	LR: 7 miles	Rest
7	E: 5 miles + 6 strides	1 mile WU; T: 3 miles; 1 mile CD	XT	1 mile WU; 4 x 400 at current 5K RP & 4 x 400 at goal 5K RP w/400 recovery; 1 mile CD	E: 3–4 miles	LR: 7–8 miles	Rest
8	E: 4 miles	1 mile WU; T: 2 x 2 miles, .5-mile recovery; 1 mile CD	XT	1 mile WU; 2 x 1000 at current 5K RP; 2 x 100 at goal 5K RP w/400 recovery; 1 mile CD	E: 3 miles	LR: 6 miles	Rest
9	Fun workout	E: 3 miles; or XT	XT	1 mile WU; 8–10 x 400 at goal 5K RP w/400 recovery; 1 mile CD	E: 3 miles	LR: 5 miles	Rest
10	E: 3 miles	1 mile WU; 2 x 400 at goal 5K RP; 4 x 200 at faster than goal 5K RP w/400 recovery; 1 mile CD	XT (light)[10]	E: 3 miles + 4 strides	E: 2–3 miles; or off[11]	5K![12]	To paraphrase our pal Kool and his Gang, celebrate good times!

1 What it says: E: 4 miles + 4 strides
What you do: Run 4 miles easy. Toward the end, along a flat stretch, run your booty off for roughly 100 meters or 30 seconds to finish one stride. Recover for roughly the same amount of distance or time, then repeat three more times.
More details: Rein yourself in during the 4 miles: It's easy to get overexcited for the strides, but stay in cruise control until it's time to rev your engine.

2 What it says:
What you do: If life collides with your training, opt out of this workout.

3 What it says: E: 3 miles; or XT
What you do: Runner's choice: Either run 3 miles easy or crosstrain. (See page 112 for suggestions.)
More details: There's no right or wrong; both options will get your body closer to the starting line.

4 What it says:
What you do: Come proverbial hell or high water, you've got to get this workout done.

5 What it says: 1 mile WU; 4 x 400 at current 5K RP w/400 recovery; 1 mile CD
What you do: Run for a mile to warm up, then run 400 meters at the pace you currently can sustain during a 5K race. Immediately following this effort, run slowly or walk for 400 meters. Repeat this fast/slow sequence for a total of four times. Trot a mile to cool down.
More details: One lap around a regulation track (read: not the dinky indoor one at your health club) = 400 meters =.25 mile. If you don't have a nearby track, use a measured quarter mile or gauge it on your wrist GPS.

6 What it says: LR: 5 miles
What you do: Hit the road or treadmill for 5 miles.
More details: Unless we tell you to go faster for part of a long run, you always want to cover the distance at a pace you could comfortably gab the whole way. (And hopefully you will, with a BRF—best running friend—by your side.)

7 What it says: Rest.
What you do: Nothing.
More details: Do we really have to tell you twice?

8 What it says: 1 mile WU; T: 2 x 1 mile, .5-mile recovery; 1 mile CD
What you do: Warm up at an easy pace for a mile. Then shift into a higher gear to run tempo pace (see page 213) for 1 mile. Take it easy for a half-mile, then crank out another faster mile, followed by a 1-mile cooldown.
More details: Tempo runs like these two 1-milers aren't all-out sprints; aim for about 75 to 85 percent power output.

9 What it says: Fun workout
What you do: Anything active your heart desires for at least 30 minutes and up to 90 minutes at a light to moderate effort. (See page 116 for suggestions.)
More details: We've all felt burned out, when running sounds as much fun as flying cross-country with a fussy baby. These wildcard workouts are shuffled into the plan to prevent ennui.

10 What it says: XT (light)
What you do: Don't push yourself too hard—or take up a new (or daredevil) sport. Now is not the time to overtax your muscles doing Zumba or break your ankle hang gliding. An easy swim, bike ride, or yoga class would be ideal. Skip doing weights.

11 What it says: E: 2–3 miles; or off
What you do: Listen to your legs—and your head. If you need to get your pre-race ya-yas out, do a light run. Otherwise, take a rest day. Both of us opt for putting our feet up.

12 What it says: 5K!
What you do: This is it—your day to bust a move.
More details: Unlike every other race distance, you don't have the luxury to ease into a 5K. Once the gun goes off, so do you. Be ready for it by running a few miles, plus a few strides (ah, your old friends), before the start.

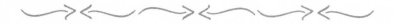

.1 ASK DIMITY

While running with friends is usually a smooth ride, even relationships built on mileage can experience a little turbulence now and then. So fasten your seat belt while I try to smooth things out.

Dear Dimity:

My best running friend just moved across the country, and I am sunk like a battleship. I have no motivation to run on. What should I do?

—To quote the Police, "I feel so lonely."

Dear So Lonely:

A split from a running buddy can be just as bad as a romantic breakup. Whenever you see your running shoes, your heart hurts; every route you drive, you remember the poignant conversations you had; every time you think of getting out there solo, you think, "But it was just so much better with her by my side."

Time passes, though, and you have to move on, which she'd want you to do. A few ways to find a new pal:

• Call a local running store or running club to find out when its group runs are. Be honest about your pace, which can be easier to do over the phone than in person. Chances are, the group runs attract all paces, but sometimes just the speedy boys show up, and you don't need to feel more left behind than you already do. On the run, pretend you're an extrovert if you're not, and see if you can't pluck a new BRF from the crowd.

• Tell people—your hairdresser, your neighbor, the mom you carpool with—that you're looking for a running buddy. They might be in the same position or know of somebody who is.

• Be bold and ask the mom who always drops her kids off at school in running clothes what she's training for and if she'd like a partner. Or ask the neighborhood woman who gardens in her Nike Tempo shorts if she's a runner.

• Enter a local half-marathon or marathon; often, longer races have Facebook pages or other virtual ways to connect, and you can post your plea there.

• Stroller Strides and Moms in Motion are two national organizations with get-'em-moving local chapters. Even if their schedule doesn't work for you on a regular basis, it's worth it to hit a class and check out the crowd to see if you can meet your match there.

• Run a race with Team in Training or another charitable organization whose cause is close to your heart. Then you and your fellow runners will have two very important things that bond you.

Dear Dimity:

I love my running friend, but she is so competitive. She drops her race times into conversations, even when I don't ask, and she always wants to know mine. How can I let her know she needs to tone it down?

—Annoyed and confused

Dear A + C:

Next time she asks about your time, go on and on about the race. You had a great race. The crowd was amazing, as was your family, who found you three times and made the cutest signs ever. You ran much stronger than you were expecting to, and can't wait to go back next year. Don't mention your time, and see if that gentle hint soaks in. If it doesn't, be more direct. "I love running with you and think these miles together are worth much more than any finishing time could indicate. I'd rather focus on our friendship than some hard, cold number."

Dear Dimity:

One of my running group members invited a new person to run with us, and I can't stand her. I'm pissed our group dynamic has been spoiled. What should I do?

—Want to trip and break her ankle

Dear Tripper:

There are two ways to deal with this. First, suck it up and find a way to either hang behind or in front of her. If your group has enough members, within a mile or two, you naturally break off into groups of two or three or, if you're so inclined, one. Nothing wrong with running on your own within the group's bubble.

If that isn't an option, and you're conflict averse, like I am, play the I-can't-run-on-our-usual-days-anymore card and bow out. You can either run solo or quietly ask one runner from the group to join you. If your splinter group ends up growing, be sure to lay out some ground rules about invitations to new members. Yes, that sounds harsh, but it's practical. Plus, I know of some book groups whose membership rules are longer than *War and Peace*.

Dear Dimity:

My friend's husband is really unsupportive of her running: He grumbles every time she asks to go for a run. She's running less and less, and I hate that. What can I do?

—Freedom ain't a state like Maine or Virginia

Dear Freedom Fighter:

Unfortunately, not much. As much as I'd like to, I can't force somebody to run, and as much as you'd like to, you can't referee somebody else's marriage. You can, however, make it as trouble-free as possible for her to get out and run. Here's how:

• Suggest that you and she run in the early morning, so that she arrives home before her household members are awake.

• Take her kids with you. Depending on the stroller situation and number of offspring, borrow a running stroller or two and alternate pushing. Or take the kids to a track, plop them in the infield with a few toys or games, and get your miles in together.

• Offer to babysit her kids at your house while she runs. Obviously, the ideal is to run together, but her running—and soaking up the confidence and strength that it brings her—would be my priority.

• When you do suggest these ideas, be as direct as possible. "We'll run tomorrow at nine o'clock at the track, so I'll pick you up at eight forty-five, okay?" so that she has less room to waffle. When you get out there together, don't talk about the husband unless she brings the topic up. Let her know you support and love her, and will do what you can to keep her moving and spending time with you.

Dear Dimity:

My friend with whom I've been training for a marathon has a stress fracture, and she's out. I've been tiptoeing around her, because I'm not sure what I should do: Do I talk about my running or the race? Or do I pretend like I'm not training anymore?

—Stressed about the stress fracture

Dear Stressed:

If you've never had an injury that prevented you from crossing the starting line, consider yourself blessed. I'll fill you in on how it feels: really, really sucky, especially for a race like a marathon, which takes up obscene amounts of your time and brain space. Combine the cramps and headaches of PMS with a bikini wax and having to put your dog to sleep, and you're coming close to how she's feeling.

You can't make it better, but you can treat her to a latte or a glass of wine (a kid-free date, preferably). As you sip, make it all about her: Ask her how she's doing, how she's filling her time, if she's caught up on all the episodes of *Big Love*, if her boss is as annoying as ever. As you well know, running isn't just a physical outlet; it's time to clear the mental fog, hang out with friends, and press the reset button. If she's a typical mom, she likely hasn't done any of that for herself since her bone cracked. Let her talk, vent, cry, and laugh while you simply listen.

After the race, get her something small like flowers (or something running related: You be the judge if that's right) and attach a note saying something like, "We'll get 'em next time."

04

THE 10K:
THE ATTAINABLE CHALLENGE

By Dimity

So those hellish 800s, back in chapter 1, are behind me. I've hit the track a few more times since then, doing about twenty more 800s, twenty 400s, and a few mile repeats spread out over various workouts. To get ready for this race, I have followed the *Run Less, Run Faster*[1] program, whose eponymous strategy recommends running less (three times a week, plus 2 crosstraining days) and faster (every run has a prescribed pace, based on your previous performance). Each week, there's a speed workout (like 800s), a tempo run (a continuous run at a demanding pace), and a longer run, which sounds kind of cruisey on paper until I realize the designated pace for the long run is actually quite a bit faster than what I naturally self-select.

While the program is definitely effective—my legs are leaner than ever, and my splits, lower than ever—it has also robbed me of my love of running. When I have to hit a certain pace for nearly every single step of every workout, a run turns into the equivalent of emptying the dishwasher, corralling my kids into bed, or picking up the dog poop in the backyard: a chore. Running is no longer an exercise in joy and me time. Still, I reluctantly finished most of the work, and I'm ready to shine my light at a 10K, a local race in early December around a small reservoir.

Mile 1 is, predictably, too fast for me. I clock in at a 7:58,[2] and know I have to settle in or I'll be doing the runner's equivalent of the collegiate walk of shame: walking at a time and place I

---

[1] It's actually a book, but writing the full title would use up most of the word allotment for this chapter. It's called *Runner's World Run Less, Run Faster: Become a Faster, Stronger Runner with the Revolutionary FIRST Training Program*, by Bill Pierce, Scott Murr, and Ray Moss. Phew.

[2] I'd rather print my weight, which is what I did in *Run Like a Mother*, than print my usual splits. But I worked hard for this one, and I want my kids to know it, so I'm recording it for posterity.

TAKE IT *From* A MOTHER
DO YOU KEEP TRACK OF RACE TIMES?

*"I write my time on the back of my bibs, which I display on
my chalkboard in my classroom. I like to see the progress
I've made, and it sets an example for my students."*

—Christy (Her 2011 goal: 1,100 kilometers [or about 684 miles], which she runs
either solo at 4:30 A.M. or occasionally with her junior high students.)

*"I keep track of my marathon times because I'm
always thinking about beating them."*

—Heather (One of her mantras, cribbed from "Intergalactic" by the
Beastie Boys: "I run the marathon till the very last mile.")

*"I've only done one race, but I keep track of every run. Maybe it's because
I need to see progress, or maybe it's just because I love spreadsheets."*

—Yeiko (Proudest running moment: when her son said he thought she could run 37 miles home from a campsite.)

*"I didn't originally, because I was much younger, thinner, and
faster—and thought I'd always be. Now I know that's not the
case, so I write them on my race bibs, which I save."*

—Alana (Doesn't know how anybody runs without doing yoga.)

*"I mentally keep track of both my most recent race time
in a distance and my PR time in that distance."*

—Kourtney (Drinks brine from the dill pickle jar if she sweats profusely during a run.)

*"Only the PRs unless it was a memorable race. I can't remember what my kids' first
words were, and I didn't write down when they lost their first teeth, so I would
feel bad if I tracked and recorded all my race times during their childhood."*

—Tricia (First ran barefoot laps around her backyard while her three girls played, then
graduated to running the cul-de-sac when they graduated to playing in the driveway.)

"Yes. I'm always trying to better my times to push myself that extra bit."

—Stephanie (Dedicates mile 20 of her marathons to the tribe of all the mother runners out there.)

PRACTICAL *Motherly* ADVICE
DOWN AND DIRTY

For moms who spend most of their days cleaning up their children, it can be therapeutic to dive into the mud themselves. These days, there are a whole category of races that involve obstacles, running, and some kind of crawl/shimmy/belly slide through a mud pit. If that's appealing to you—and it's totally understandable if it's not—here are some ways to make sure your race is as dirty as possible.

9 Put together a great costume, if you're so inclined. Tutus, neon spandex, leotards, fish nets, fake fur, body paint, even a cropped wedding dress (yup, we've seen it) all work well and will put you in the spirit. If donning tulle and sparkles is a little much, at least come up with a great name if you're doing a team race in pairs: Dirty Girlz, Mud Mamas, Partners in Grime, Dirty Divas, or, of course, Badass Mother Runners.

9 Do not sport any jewelry—especially not your diamond-studded engagement ring.

9 Do not bring any electronics—especially not your Garmin.

9 Wear your oldest running shoes. If you retired them 2 months ago and now use them for walking your hound, they're perfect. Don't fret about the effect of running 3 or 6 miles in expired kicks: You're most likely not going to be motoring at race pace.

shouldn't be. I slow down a little but still have enough pep in my legs to pass people. I'm usually music-less in races, and, as a result, often tune into the breathing around me and use that to gauge my effort. Am I a bigger huffer and puffer than the guy next to me? Then I'll just chill. Am I hardly exhaling, compared with Mrs. Gasp over there? Then turn it up, sister.

Today, I am astonished at the heavy breathing going on around me. My lungs feel as full as a freshly inflated helium balloon. I pump it up another notch. I pass a woman in a Timex jersey (read: she's on a sponsored team) and I think, *I'll feel stupid when she gets me again, but at least I'll have one short-lived moment of glory from running less and running faster.*

Despite my Breathalyzer tests and somewhat speedy legs, I do my best to stay controlled until the halfway point. A 10K is the perfect distance to really learn how to pace yourself and run a smart

9 Mark your gear. In races involving a bike, tie a helium-filled balloon to the seat so you can spot it easily in transition areas. Note: the seat, *not* the handlebars, or you'll be viewing the racecourse through helium-filled lenses.

9 Confine yourself: The tighter your clothes, the better. Anything draping or gaping is an invitation for dirt to get into places you'd rather not have it.

9 Secure your gear as best you can. Firmly tie, then double-knot, your shoelaces *and* the drawstring in your tights or shorts. If the race involves lots of running through muck, consider wrapping duct tape around your shoes (after you put them on!) to keep them from getting sucked off your feet by the gunk.

9 Bring a stash of old towels. Most finish areas will have a hose-you-off system, which usually gets you to a level of clean akin to your 4-year-old washing his own face; the apparent spots of filth are gone, but a layer of grime lingers. Towels multitask well: You can use one as a screen when you change into fresh clothes for the drive home, then lay others on your car seat as a barrier between you and your car's upholstery.

9 Yuk—or is it yuck?—it up along the course. Just be sure to keep your mouth closed when you're crawling through the mud.

race. A middle child parked between the guns-blazing 5K and the don't-go-gonzo half-marathon, the 10K requires you to practice both self-confidence and self-restraint. At a little more than 6 miles, it's a great trial size of racing. Did you get a little too broad chested and shoot your wad? The finish line is only 2—not 6—miles away. Or are you a little too unsure of yourself around mile 3? You still have another few miles to prove to your legs that you're in charge. What's more, the race neatly divides up into two 5Ks, so there's no room for confusion in pace strategy. For the first half, you go slower than you think you should; for the second, faster.

Taking my own advice, I find myself at the 4-mile mark, with splits still averaging under 8:20. I also find myself in quite a bit of pain. My legs aren't really interested in running faster anymore, but I have simply trained too little and too fast, figuratively speaking, to let myself flake.

So I revert to my best mental strategy for passing time on the road: breaking up the race into bites as small as I'd slice up hot dogs for a preschooler. I subdivide the remaining distance into twenty-two tenths of a mile. (SBS sometimes calls me Rain Man for good reason.) During the first ten mental segments, I probably look at my Garmin thirty times. At mile 5—twelve more pieces to go—two women running side by side pass me on the concrete path, and I decide I will stay as close to them as I can. In my mind, I am drafting off them, but at a head taller than both of them, I am really just sponging up their momentum. I crack out another (barely) sub-8 minute. *Me? Click off a sub-8 for the last mile of a 10K?*

"Excuse me," I gasp to the two of them when I spy the finish line, passing them on the left as I pick it up to a sprint. Nope, not a typo: a sprint after already running 6 miles. I clear the two gal pals and cross in 50:20ish, good enough for fifth place in my age group.

As I hope you know, I'm usually not somebody who waxes on about my times and race results. But that 10K was the most surreal race I've ever had. Honestly, it was like an out-of-body experience, like I was running a perfect race I had visualized, if I ever actually took the time to sit down, focus, and mentally rehearse my race. (I only shave my legs every 4 weeks, so it goes without saying, I've never practiced visualization.) I felt so strong and so confident; I knew when I passed people, I was putting distance between me and them, not just eking by them and beginning my typical game of pass/be passed/pass/be passed. (Minus Ms. Timex, of course. As far as I'm concerned, anybody in a sponsored jersey can come back to bite me at any time.)

I know this race will stand for all eternity as my 10K PR. I was proud to have run it and amazed I had a real kick, yet I was even more glad to return to my regularly scheduled running. Running (a wee bit) more, and definitely running slower.

10K: FINISH IT

"A 10K is great because I don't feel like I have to gun it, but it's still over fairly quickly."

—KIRSTEN

Best for: Somebody tackling the distance for the first time—or coming back from injury.

Physical Prereq: Chicas ready for this challenge should be able to run 3 or 4 miles comfortably. It's a good idea to have completed a 5K race and have a few months of consistent running logged on your legs, but if you're a newbie to speedwork, no worries: We'll ease you into it.

Plan Overview: This 10-weeker stretches out your long runs to 7 miles to build the requisite stamina and confidence to cover 6.2 miles, while also introducing some speedier workouts. We're not asking you to bust a move too often, but we know you're up for the occasional challenge, right?

10K: Finish It

Quick Key:

= Bail if necessary.

= Bailing is not an option.

CD = Cooldown
E = Easy
I = Interval
LR = Long run

WU = Warm-up
XT = Crosstrain
Z = Zone (see page 118 for definitions)

WEEK	MONDAY	TUESDAY	WEDNESDAY	THURSDAY	FRIDAY	SATURDAY	SUNDAY
1	E: 3 miles + 4 strides[1]	Fun workout[2]	E: 3 miles + 4 strides	XT[3]	[4] E: 3 miles	[5] LR: 4 miles[6]	Rest[7]
2	E: 3 miles + 6 strides	E: 2–3 miles; or XT	3 miles as 10 min. WU; I: 6 x 1 min. in Z4 w/2–3 min. recovery; 10 min. CD[8]	XT	E: 3 miles	LR: 5 miles	Rest
3	E: 3 miles + 8 strides	E: 3 miles; or XT	3.5 miles as 10 min. WU; I: 3 x 4 min. in Z3 w/2–3 min. recovery; 10 min. CD	XT	E: 3 miles	LR: 6 miles	Rest

10K: Finish It *continued*

4	E: 3 miles + 4 strides	Fun workout	3.5 miles as 10 min. WU; I: 6 x 2 min. in Z4 w/2 min. recovery; 10 min. CD	XT	E: 3 miles	LR: 5 miles	Rest
5	E: 3 miles + 6 strides	E: 3 miles; or XT	4 miles as 10 min. WU; I: 4 x 4 min. in Z3 w/3 min. recovery; 10 min. CD	XT	E: 3 miles	LR: 6 miles	Rest
6	E: 3 miles + 8 strides	E: 3 miles; or XT	4 miles as 10 min. WU; I: 8–10 x 1 min. in Z4 w/2 min. recovery; 10 min. CD	XT	E: 3 miles	LR: 7 miles	Rest
7	E: 3 miles + 8 strides	Fun workout	E: 3–4 miles	XT	E: 3 miles	LR: 5 miles	Rest
8	E: 3 miles + 8 strides	E: 3 miles; or XT	4–5 miles as 10 min. WU; I: 3 x 5 min. in Z3 w/3 min. recovery; 10 min. CD	XT	E: 3 miles	LR: 6–7 miles	Rest
9	E: 3 miles + 6 strides	E: 3 miles; or XT	3–4 miles as 10 min. WU; I: 8 x 2 min. in Z4 w/2 min. recovery; 10 min. CD	XT	E: 3 miles	LR: 4–5 miles	Rest
10	3 miles as 10 min. WU; I: 4 x 1 min. in Z4 w/1 min. recovery; 10 min. recovery	E: 2–3 miles; or XT	E: 3 miles + 4–6 strides	Rest	E: 20–30 min. + 2–4 strides	10K![9]	Sleep in.

1 What it says: E: 3 miles + 4 strides

What you do: Three miles at a chatable pace, then shift gears to do four strides. How to stride: On flat ground, incrementally increase your speed until you're going 90 to 95 percent max, and go about 100 meters or 30 seconds. Recover as needed between each souped-up effort.

More details: Finishing an easy run with strides reminds your body how to move quickly and efficiently.

2 What it says: Fun workout

What you do: Anything your heart desires—as long as it gets it pumping faster. Could be playing touch football with your neighbors or bodysurfing. (See page 116 for ideas.)

More details: Use this workout to press your reset button.

3 What it says: XT

What you do: Thirty to 60 minutes of weight training, yoga, cycling, swimming, Pilates: any crosstraining activity that strengthens your muscles and/or cardio system while giving your body a break from running's repetitive pounding.

4 What it says:

What you do: Whether it's after a night of constant interruptions (is *anyone* in your house not hacking?) or the day before a big run, you can skip this workout, guilt free.

More details: These workouts will be either a shorter easy run or a crosstraining day. Missing one or the other occasionally will have the least amount of impact on your overall fitness and race preparedness.

5 What it says:

What you do: Don't let anything—not work deadlines, whiny kids, or the sniffles—get in the way of this workout.

More details: Do what you can to avoid missing your interval workouts and long runs. Both endurance and speed are important elements of a successful 10K finish.

6 What it says: LR: 4 miles

What you do: Trot through 4 miles at a comfortable pace that you could sustain for much longer than 4 miles.

TAKE IT *From* A MOTHER
DO YOU BUY PICTURES OF YOURSELF IN A RACE?

"Nope, but I always check them out and am frustrated that it looks like I have both feet on the ground."

—JULIE (Best running memory: crossing the line of the 100th Boston Marathon: "Tears still come to my eyes when retelling my race experience.")

"I bought a picture of me crossing the finish line in a half-marathon at 1:59. My husband ran in with me, so he's in the picture smiling at me while I have my arms up and a huge smile."

—KELLY (Entertains herself on runs by turning mailbox numbers into math equations, e.g., for 246, she thinks 2 + 4 = 6.)

"Yes, I always buy at least one, because I need proof I was there and did it."

—KERI (First race, a 5K, was with her daughter; second race, a half-marathon, was with her mom.)

"No, but my local running store does a lot of races, and they provide free pictures."

—CAROL (Her dream running date: her hubby, not wearing a shirt. "He's sexy as all get out but hates going shirtless. Shorts that show off his nice butt would be cool, too.")

"I bought pictures from my half-marathon. It felt like a virgin experience that I needed to own, even if the pictures sucked. The other races, I resisted."

—KRISTI (Spends more money on running clothes than regular clothes: "I splurge on the bottoms and spend a little less on the tops.")

"I bought one from the first marathon. I look at other race pictures to check out my form and make corrections later. I don't buy them, though. Maybe I would if I looked happy instead of like I am going to kill somebody."

—KELLY (Forcing her whole family to come to her next marathon, where she'll assign them positions and give them cowbells.)

> *"No. My husband has a great camera with action mode, so we take our own shots, and they turn out awesome."*
>
> —ALICE (Fave crosstraining: housework. "There is always lots to do.")

> *"Not until I look decent in one of them."*
>
> —MARY-GLEN (Date night is a run with her husband: "We get to talk to each other, and are not spending money on an average dinner or movie.")

7 What it says: Rest
What you do: Give your body a well-deserved break.

8 What it says: 3 miles as 10 min. WU; I: 6 x 1 min. in Z4 w/2–3 min. recovery; 10 min. CD
What you do: Cover 3 miles by warming up for 10 minutes, then ratcheting up your speed for 1 minute—aim to get in Zone 4—then recover for 2 to 3 minutes. Finish with 10 minutes of easier running.
More details: Yes, a lot of looking at your watch, but this workout will fly by.

9 What it says: 10K!
What you do: Remind yourself of all the work that got you to this point, then let your effort shine on the racecourse.
More details: No sugarcoating: You'll feel taxed about 4 miles in, but the finish line will come sooner than you and your legs think.

10K: OWN IT

"I'm a 10K girl. When you put effort into the training, you feel like a million bucks at the end of a race."

—MEGAN

Best for: A runner who has prior 10K and 5K race experience and wants to bang out a solid 10K effort—or PR.

Physical Prereq: You should be able to complete a 6-mile run and have experience turning up the pace. If you haven't, you might want to own a 5K race before taking on this one.

Plan Overview: Ten weeks will take you to a rip-roarin' fast 10K; along the way, you'll build your cardiovascular base with long runs, hit some hills to up your strength, sprint to get your speed up, and hone in on your race pace. Don't worry: It's not as tough as it sounds.

1 What it says: E: 3 miles; or XT
What you do: Run 3 relaxed miles or crosstrain for 30 to 60 minutes, depending how much bounce is in your step.
More details: Most weeks have 3 days with choices. I—Dimity—would probably choose to run one day (Mondays), crosstrain one day (Wednesdays), and rest the third day (Fridays). SBS would run two of the three, and XT the other.

2 What it says:
What you do: Get it done, sister.
More details: Each week, there's one workout critical to you owning the 10K. This is the one.

3 What it says: 4 miles as 10 min. WU; I: 12 x 1 min. in Z4 w/1 min. recovery; 10 min. CD
What you do: Warm up for 10 minutes, then start in on some intervals: Run 1 minute in Zone 4 (this is *hard* work), run easy/walk for 1 minute. Repeat nine more times. Cool down for 10 minutes. Your total mileage will end up around 4 miles.
More details: Four miles is an estimate. Come in at 3 or 5? No problem. Don't go all high maintenance on the numbers.

10K: Own It

Quick Key:

= Bail if necessary.

= Bailing is not an option.

CD = Cooldown

E = Easy
H = Hills
I = Interval
LR = Long run
RP = Race pace (see page 105 to determine yours)

T = Tempo (see page 213 for definition)
WU = Warm-up
XT = Crosstrain
Z = Zone (see page 118 for definitions)

WEEK	MONDAY	TUESDAY	WEDNESDAY	THURSDAY	FRIDAY	SATURDAY	SUNDAY
1	E: 3 miles; or XT[1]	[2] 4 miles as 10 min. WU; I: 12 x 1 min. in Z4 w/1 min. recovery; 10 min. CD[3]	[4] E: 3 miles; or XT	1–2 mile WU; T: 1 mile; 1–2 mile CD[5]	Rest; or XT[6]	LR: 6 miles[7]	Rest[8]
2	E: 3 miles; or XT	1–2 mile WU; H: 8 x 1 min. in Z4; 1–2 mile CD[9]	Fun work-out[10]	E: 4 miles	Rest; or XT	LR: 7 miles	Rest
3	E: 3 miles; or XT	1–2 mile WU; 4 x 800 w/400 recovery; 1–2 mile CD[11]	E: 3 miles; or XT	1–2 mile WU; T: 2 x 1 mile w/.5-mile recovery; 1–2 mile CD	Rest; or XT	LR: 8 miles	Rest
4	E: 3 miles; or XT	4 miles as 10 min. warm-up; I: 5 x 3 min. in Z3 w/2 min. recovery; 10 min. CD	E: 3 miles; or XT	E: 4 miles	Rest; or XT	LR: 6 miles, 10 min. strong fin-ish[12]	Rest
5	E: 3 miles; or XT	1–2 mile WU; H: 5 x 2 min. in Z4; 1–2 mile CD	E: 3 miles; or XT	1–2 mile WU; T: 2 miles; 1–2 miles CD	Rest; or XT	LR: 8–9 miles	Rest
6	E: 3 miles; or XT	1–2 mile WU; 3 x 1000 at RP w/400 recovery; 1–2 mile CD[13]	Fun workout	E: 4–5 miles	Rest; or XT	LR: 7 miles, 15 min. strong finish	Rest

10K: Own It *continued*

7	E: 3 miles; or XT	4 miles as 10 min. WU; I: 5 x 2 min. in Z4 w/1 min. recovery; 10 min. CD	E: 3 miles; or XT	1–2 mile WU; T: 2 x 1 mile + RP: 1 x 1 mile, all w/400 recovery; 1–2 mile CD[14]	Rest; or XT	LR: 8–9 miles	Rest
8	E: 3 miles; or XT	1–2 mile WU; H: 5 x 2:30 min. in Z3–4; 1–2 mile CD	Fun workout	E: 4–5 miles	Rest; or XT	LR: 9–10 miles	Rest
9	E: 3 miles + 6 strides	E: 3 miles; or XT	3–4 miles as 10 min. WU; I: 8 x 2 min. in Z4 w/2 min. recovery; 10 min. CD	XT	E: 3 miles	LR: 4–5 miles	Rest
10	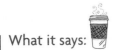 3 miles as 10 min. WU; I: 4 x 1 min. in Z4 w/1 min. recovery; 10 min. recovery	E: 2–3 miles; or XT	E: 3 miles + 4–6 strides	Rest	E: 20–30 min. + 2–4 strides	10K![15]	Eat a great brunch.

4 What it says:

What you do: Give yourself a choice: Do you want to stay or go?

More details: Once a week, there's a workout that is optional. It won't blow your finish time to skip it, as long as you're diligent with the other ones.

5 What it says: 1–2 mile WU; T: 1 mile; 1–2 mile CD

What you do: Enjoy a nice 1- to 2-mile warm-up, crank it up a notch for a mile at tempo pace, then cool that body down for another 1 to 2 miles.

6 What it says: Rest; or XT

What you do: Had a relatively tranquil week? Crosstrain. Ready to jump off a cliff? Rest.

7 What it says: LR: 6 miles
What you do: Run for 6 consecutive miles at a pace that leaves you energized for the rest of the day.

8 What it says: Rest.
What you do: Don't work up a sweat today. Or at least not until you hook up with your SO.

9 What it says: 1–2 mile WU; H: 8 x 1 min. in Z4; 1–2 mile CD
What you do: Warm up your little booty for 1 to 2 miles, and end at the base of a moderate hill that is at least a minute long. (As the intervals grow, the length of the hill needs to, as well.) Run up the hill at a steady pace, keeping your effort as even as possible so you don't peter out at the top. Run slowly or walk to the bottom and begin again; do eight climbs total. Finish with a 1- to 2-mile cooldown on flattish ground.

More details: If you live in the Sunshine State or another hill-deprived area, find a bridge, empty parking garage, or hit the treadmill at a 4 to 6 percent incline. You don't want it so steep you're crawling on all fours, but make sure it's a challenging grade. Live among the hillbillies? Mix up the hills you use from one workout to the next.

10 What it says: Fun workout
What you do: Put a smile on your face, flip to page 116, pick a workout, and don't stop smiling until the workout is done. (And, yes, we're watching.)

11 What it says: 1–2 mile WU; 4 x 800 w/400 recovery; 1–2 mile CD
What you do: Run 1 to 2 miles as a warm-up, either at the track or to a track. Run an 800 (two times around) at race pace, then jog or walk a 400 (once around). Repeat three more times. Cool down with 1 to 2 miles.

More details: If you don't have a specific number in mind, race-pace effort is a notch up from tempo (roughly 20 seconds faster), or about 85 percent of all you've got to give. These runs teach you to run through fatigue. (And you thought the only learning you did these days was helping your fourth-grader with long division.)

12 What it says: LR: 6 miles, 10 min. strong finish
What you do: Head out for 6 miles, and for the last 10 minutes, bump up your effort a notch so that you're hitting a tempoish pace.
More details: Do your best to speed it up, but if you're having a crappy run, hanging in there—and just not letting yourself slow down—is an acceptable definition of "strong finish."

13 What it says: 1–2 mile WU; 3 x 1000 at RP w/400 recovery; 1–2 mile CD
What you do: Ease into your workout by running 1 to 2 miles, ending at a track. Run 1,000 meters (2.5 times around a track or .62 miles) at your projected 10K race pace, then recover by running once around the track slowly. Run two more 1,000-meter repeats with 400-meter recovery, then run 1 or 2 miles to cool down.

14 What it says: 1–2 mile WU; T: 2 x 1 mile + RP: 1 x 1 mile, all w/400 recovery; 1–2 mile CD
What you do: Usual warm-up, then run 1 mile at tempo pace, recover for 400 meters (or .25 mile), run another mile at tempo pace, recover for 400 meters, then finish with 1 mile at race pace. Thank your legs for their awesome effort, then finish with a 1- to 2-mile cooldown.
More details: I—Dimity—would skip the final 400-meter recovery and head straight into the cooldown. Because that's how I roll.

15 What it says: 10K!
What you do: Race for 6.2 miles of pure ecstasy! Or something like that.
More details: A solid PR strategy: Divide the race into thirds. For the first 2 miles, aim to hit your goal pace. The second 2 miles, you will most likely pass all the runners who went out too fast. Use that as a mental boost and pick people off, as you maintain your pace and avoid the thoughts of slowing down that are screaming for attention right about now. Know the last 2.2 miles are going to be uncomfy. Staying mentally strong is key in this final stretch. Hang on to people in front of you and imagine being pulled or slung past them. Do all you can to maintain or even surpass your pace in that final mile. Last .2, pretend you have balls, and slam them into the wall.

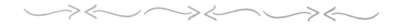

.1 FROM ELATION TO EXHAUSTION: A TEAM RELAY
By **Dimity**

Relay races started in 1982 with a few ragtag runners on the bucolic back roads of Oregon, doing the Hood to Coast (now dubbed, aptly enough, "the mother of all relays"). They've since blossomed into a too-legit-to-quit race category. Typically, teams of a dozen runners, single sex or coed, progress from scenic Point A to lovely Point B with each runner doing three legs that total roughly 14 to 20 miles. Sounds amazing, but running double digits and staying up for nearly a day straight can be a little taxing. To wit:

5 P.M. Wednesday [44 hours before start]
Scramble to find new 12th member of team to replace the mother runner whose kid just broke her arm at the playground. She still wants to go, but her husband isn't sure he can take care of a kid with a broken wing and her two siblings. "What does he think you have to do while he's at work all week?" asks the captain, silently assuring herself the husband must have some redeeming qualities.

1 P.M. Thursday
Two members hit up Costco for everything they ogle but never buy when shopping for their families. Huge bags of sea-salt chips (considered healthy food: salt, lost through sweat, is actually a necessity, right?); 50 small bags of Mrs. Field's Cookies; a tub of chocolate-covered pretzels; enough licorice for a YMCA camp for a week; a gallon of Advil. For good measure, they throw in some bananas, bagels, and sports drinks.

11 P.M. Thursday
You attempt to clean out your Sienna, which will soon be one of the official team vans. Spelling tests from 6 months ago, old milk boxes (so *that's* what that smell was), and random Legos all go in the trash. If nothing else, you rationalize, at least you'll have a clean car in exchange for running (gulp) 18 miles.

9 A.M. Friday
Twelve moms, all used to being micromanagers, put on their supervisor hats and attempt to cram in twelve bags of gear, a couple sleeping bags and pillows, two tarps, the Costco-run sustenance, and a water jug resembling an orange Michelin Man into what now feels like two terribly small vans.

1 P.M. Friday

Start! Thanks to a visiting sister-in-law, who is training for the NYC Marathon and jumped in to be Leg 8 runner, all twelve runners head to the start to cheer on the runner of the first leg. Lots of pictures, lots of laughs from everybody in their matching "Tough Mothers" tanks and black skirts. Excitement—and nervous energy—course through your veins. As the vans pass by your runner, you hang out the window and scream like you're a teenager seeing Justin Bieber.

1:45 P.M. Friday

First handoff. Again, everybody enthusiastically gets out of the van. Go team! High fives all around.

5 P.M. Friday

Contemplate an apple but break out the Red Vines instead, rationalizing the high sugar content qualifies as carbo-loading.

5:25 P.M. Friday

Your first leg: 5.4 miles. A few uphills, but it feels so good to run after sitting in a van for 5 hours. Cakewalk.

7:20 P.M. Friday

You climb out to cheer on the final handoff of this series of six legs, and those hills, which had seemed so mild mannered, are reverberating through your legs with every step you take.

8:40 P.M. Friday

You poll your van mates about what to do during the first big break while Van 2 runners are blazing through the course. Despite your hard but tactful lobbying, your suggestion to grab drive-through then some shut-eye gets voted down in favor of a sit-down meal at Olive Garden.

12:25 A.M. Saturday

Hustle teammates to the van—you're worried you'll miss the handoff with Van 2 in the dark.

12:40 A.M. Saturday

Spy your first nighttime runners. Get chills from envisioning yourself out there running—and from the 48-degree night air.

1:15 A.M. Saturday

The skuzzy camping feeling has set in. You deeply regret the endless-breadsticks choice, which meant no time to shower at the team captain's house. Judging from the stench wafting off your teammate who is copiloting as you drive, you must be smelling rank, too. Vow to brush your teeth and wipe your pits at the next transition.

2:35 A.M. Saturday

Consider drinking a bottled Frappuccino to revive, but the mere thought makes you throw up a little in your mouth. The flat of them at Costco had looked so appetizing.

3:55 A.M. Saturday

Your second leg: 7 miles. Wearing a headlamp and a sweaty reflective vest and carrying a glow stick in each hand, you look like a Christmas tree. Despite the cool night air, your legs start to cooperate after a mile. Birds start to twitter; it's beginning to feel like morning instead of nighttime. Rejoice as you contemplate how amazingly different this run is from the basement-treadmill ones you are often forced to do during your toddler's naps. *There's nothing I'd rather do in the predawn darkness than run 7 miles*, you think to yourself. Until you hit more hills, which you don't see until you're at the bottom of them, looking up. *Why do my legs have all the hills?*

4:55 A.M. Saturday

You know it's antisocial, but you doze off instead of getting out of the van to cheer on and hand water to a teammate halfway through her (way-less-hilly-than-your) leg.

8 A.M. Saturday

The smell coming off the two Porta-Potties at the transition is so revolting, you decide to squat by the side of the road and realize you've forgotten the TP, which isn't as pristine as it was a day ago. Drip dry, or so you think, until you stand up and dribble all over your inner thigh. Contemplate sharing anecdote with a teammate but realize it may only be funny to you—or at the end of the race. Anybody know where the Purell is?

8:35 A.M. Saturday

Spy the van of the Fairfield Fairies, a team of tutu-clad 20-something women runners your team has been jockeying with since the early stages of the race. The urge to overtake them is less compelling than it was, oh, 19 hours ago. (Is that really all it's been?)

9 A.M. Saturday

Tally off what you've eaten so far: flavorless, too-salty spaghetti puttanesca at the O. Garden; half an Egg McMuffin (you would've eaten the whole thing, but it fell into a puddle at a transition area . . . the 5-second rule couldn't apply); four bags of mini Mrs. Fields; three bottles of Powerade; a PB&J; at least fifteen Red Vines; two bananas; five handfuls of Fritos, and, to make sure you had enough fuel to finish your legs, two gels while running. Decide you've consumed far more calories than you've burned running.

9:10 A.M. Saturday

After the handoff with Van 2, you navigate the now-dust-caked Sienna into a massive field that resembles a Civil War battlefield, if fleece hoodies and running shoes had been standard issue for Union troops. Scope out a secluded spot—a relative term when you're talking 213 decorated vans and 1,200-plus runners—to spread out your tarp and sleeping bag. Pull on an eye pillow to block out the sun and hook your hand over your ear to block the noise of other racers having the Hershey squirts in the nearby wooded area.

1:15 P.M. Saturday

Last leg: 3.6 miles. Relive the McMuffin as it reappears as you hit yet *another* hill on your final leg, which is, thankfully, mostly flat and downhill. All good, except it starts to rain.

2:00 P.M. Saturday

Go through all your clothes—you thought you brought enough for a week—and realize you don't have anything that is both clean *and* dry. Settle for your sweat-stained team tank and a random black fleece you found stashed in the backseat along with McDonald's wrappers, used Kleenex, a stash of celebrity gossip mags (score!), and a smooshed bran muffin. Your kids are less messy than your friends.

2:15 P.M. Saturday

Forget dancing by the side of the road or flirting with the Midnight Cowboys team of young'uns from the University of Texas. Try to sleep in the van. Get so annoyed by a teammate's high-pitched voice you put on your iPod, but Lady Gaga's "Edge of Glory," which got you so fired up yesterday afternoon, doesn't really have the lullaby vibe you need. More like "Edge of Insanity."

5:42 P.M. Saturday

Finish! Big group hug, lots of pics (that will never make it past Facebook), and a few tears. We did this! Vow you'll *definitely* do another relay next year.

05

THE HALF-MARATHON:
THE SWEET SPOT

By Dimity

When Sarah and I go to expos to spread the Another Mother Runner love at races that feature both a half-marathon and a marathon, I'm always nosy about what distance people are running when they come to our table. A typical response from another mother runner: "Oh, just the half-marathon."

I get a little preachy at this answer. "Don't put 'just' in that sentence," I say, more serious than my joking tone indicates. "Thirteen point one miles is not an insignificant distance. You're not running *just* the half-marathon. You're running *the* half-marathon."

Part of my attitude comes from being weary of women, including myself, constantly belittling our running and other accomplishments: "I *just* have two kids." "I *just* work part time." "I *just* scrapbook and blog." When's the last time you heard a man minimize his accomplishments? Ladies, own the race—and all the other work you do.

But I also get all uppity because the half-marathon is my favorite distance.[1] Like Netflix, nostir natural peanut butter, and plastic sheets to protect mattresses from pee, the half-marathon, at its core, is simply a great invention for mothers—and especially mother runners. It requires a serious commitment (read: lots of alone, or BRF, time), but doesn't monopolize your life like its bigger sister, the marathon, can and usually does. For newer runners stepping up from a shorter distance, the intimidation factor of a halfsie is significantly less than the full monty, but in my mind the rewards are on par, if not better. You still get to say the word *marathon* when somebody asks you what race you're doing. You still cross into double-digit territory mileage-wise. You still have to bust out of your

---

[1] I'm not the only one who hearts 13.1 miles. If Another Mother Runner had a theme race, it would be the half-marathon. According to Running USA, the corrals are filling up with our tribe, as 820,000 women, or 59 percent of total race finishers, crossed the finish line of a half-marathon in 2010, a sixfold increase since 1995.

neighborhood-route box. But you don't put yourself as close to the edge of injury, running burnout, and general exhaustion.

In other words, training for and running 13.1 miles is simultaneously achievable and challenging; elevating and pleasantly draining; confidence building and self-doubt invoking. A half-marathon makes me feel, mile by mile, gloriously human—and not just like a mother who alternates between giving praise and time-outs.

As I mentioned, 13.1 miles is not an insignificant distance, and, being a genetically ungifted runner, I've learned I can't flake on training. I "ran" one half after a training regimen during which my longest pre-race run was 9 miles and my adherence to weekday runs would not have earned any gold stars. I eked out those last 4.1 miles, but I felt like I was hauling two 65-pound rocks around. (Oh, I was: They were my dead legs.) Even worse, I was full-marathon sore the next day. Toilet seat hover, backward down the stairs, no kids allowed in the vicinity of my lap, the whole deal. I promised myself I wouldn't do that again.

So when I've got a half-marathon in my crosshairs, those do-I-*really*-need-to-run reservations that seem as much a part of my early morning ritual as listening to the weather on the radio get (mostly) pushed aside. I've got to focus and stay honest with my runs, especially with the long ones, the backbone of any half-marathon plan. Most of the training runs are lengthy enough to make me buzz with accomplishment for the rest of the day, but they don't suck the life out of me, like the loooooong 18- or 20-milers a marathon requires. (If you groove on those, like SBS does, more power to you. I most definitely do not.) With an 11-miler, I can be out the door at 6:30 on a Saturday morning, home by 8:30, grab a bagel, shower, stretch a bit, bask in the glow that I just ran 11 miles, get to Ben's T-ball by 9:30, and still be relatively good to go for the rest of the day. I may need to go to bed earlier than normal or take a nap, but where's the harm in that?

The other advantage of the half-marathon long run: When I'm training properly, I often come close to, or exceed, race-day distance, so any doubts about whether I can go the distance are quelled before race day. My confidence increases accordingly. (Yes, after 20 years of running, one would think a half-marathon is a no-brainer for me, but it's not, especially after stints of having kids, being injured, or otherwise slacking. Much to my chagrin, there are no savings accounts in running.) Marathon training plans, which often top out at 20 or 22 miles, require a leap of faith to get to 26.2 miles on race day. While I understand the less-is-more rationale—the training, taper, race atmosphere, and sheer determination will get you there—my life is full of enough uncertainty as it is. Call me conservative, but I like to know I can finish what I start.

TAKE IT *From* A MOTHER
WHAT DO YOU CARRY ON TRAINING RUNS?

"I have a Ricola Honey Lemon Echinacea lozenge under my tongue on every run."

—ALISON (Post-race meal: "Anything with calories. Butter and sugar are always welcome.")

"I used to carry nothing. Now I carry my phone, at my husband's insistence, because, once early in tree-pollen season, I forgot to take my allergy meds. I swelled up like the Stay Puft Marshmallow Man from Ghostbusters and had to be rescued by the kind people at my kid's school."

—CLAIRE (Her 3-year-old's reaction to a picture of a Memorial Day parade: "Look, it's a race, Mom.")

"For short runs, I take only music, but for longer runs I add in ChapStick, gummi bears, and water."

—SUE (Refuses to buy a Garmin for fear she would become obsessed with splits and times. *Note: She's right. She would.*)

"I started carrying my cell phone so I could snap photos of deer, antelope, coyotes, and foxes I see on my run. I want to be able to brag to my friends who are running in traffic back in civilization."

—CHANDRA (Uses dailymile to train virtually with her best friend, who is 2,000 miles away.)

"Water belt, cell phone, gel, $10, pepper spray, and whistle. Of course, the pepper spray and whistle are securely tucked inside, so it would require significant fumbling in an emergency."

—JILL (When running on trails, she imagines she's on a trail in Forks, Washington, and Edward or Jacob—the good guys from *Twilight*—swoop in to save her from Laurent, the bad vampire.)

"Nothing extra."

—NEITA (Best motivation: gratefulness that she can run.)

"An iPod, but sometimes I run without it. Does a good attitude count?"

—CATEY (Fave running wardrobe item: a self-made zebra skirt.)

Run LIKE THIS MOTHER
SHOULD I STAY OR SHOULD I GO?

By Sarah

To me, running a race with a friend ranks right up there with sleeping in and eating homegrown to-matoes as one of life's great, simple pleasures. But it's not as easy as it sounds: Races can be crowded, paces can vary, goals can be different, and expectations can shift. Heck, even having to pee can be the deciding factor, like it was for Sheila and me in the 2010 Portland Marathon.

At several previous marathons, I'd missed hitting my goal time by less than 2 minutes—basi-cally the amount of time it takes to duck into a Porta-Potty, void my bladder, wrestle my sweaty capris back up, and rejoin the race. I wasn't going to let that happen again. So I vowed to pee in my pants if the urge to purge struck during the race. (At the start of the race, I practiced peeing during the national anthem to be certain I could pull it off without pulling it down, so to speak. Trust me on this one: It's tough, as an adult, to piss in your pants. My REI capris absorbed most of the odorless pee, which was mainly just filtered-through-my-kidneys water I'd sucked down 2 hours prior. And, it was pouring rain, so the torrent of raindrops served as a natural flush.) Sheila, however, wasn't down with my plan. Wearing shorts, she insisted she would stop along the course if the need arose.

And it did, for her, around mile 4. Although we had the same time goal, we'd agreed pre-race we were each going to run our own race. So when she stopped to use the loo, I trotted off without any guilt. I wished her well and urged her to catch up with me posthaste. (I ended up making our goal; she, alas, missed it.)

Six weeks later, at the Philadelphia half-marathon, I was more conflicted about leaving my buddy behind. This time my running companion was my BFF, Courtenay, who lives 3,000 miles away from me (unlike Portlander Sheila, who I can run with any day of the week). I had hoped to pull Court to a sub-2:00 half-marathon, but after 3 miles of what I considered an ease-into-it pace, Court gasped out, "I can't go this fast for 10 more miles." We had discussed beforehand the merits of staying together versus running our separate ways, and Court had let me know, in no uncertain terms, she'd be ticked at me if I slowed down to stay with her. Having known, and loved, each other since high school, we don't have any doublespeak or code: Court said she wanted me to run ahead, and I knew she sincerely meant it. I sped up, shouting out a reminder of our already-agreed-upon, post-race meeting place.

(Dimity chiming in here: As the one who is often the leavee, not the leaver, I'm 100 percent with Courtenay on this one. The only thing worse than feeling like you're slowing somebody down is to feel forced to maintain a pace you know is too fast.)

Before I share some advice, please know I am capable of running an entire race by my friend's side. Most recently I helped Molly, the mom we carpool to school with, set her 13.1-mile PR. Plus, Molly, not me, pulled ahead a quarter-mile from the finish. (You go, Mol!) She crossed the line 14 seconds before I did, and I couldn't have been more proud of her accomplishment.

PRE-RACE

- Have a candid conversation with your friend about expectations and goals. If she's looking to hustle in the race, whereas you're looking to boogie the night before, perhaps the race will be your alone time during a girls' race weekend.

- Make a playlist and share it with your BRF. Whether you run together or apart, you'll be united with your tunes.

- Decide where to convene after the finish. Many races, especially marathons or bigger races, often have a racers-only area after the finish line you can't reenter once you leave. If you can, figure out a place in that restricted area to meet, as there will be runner replenishment available (fruit, bottled water, bagels, yogurt, candy bars, chocolate milk, you name it). Also, set a generous time, like an hour after you predict the slower person will finish, after which you meet at your car or hotel, so one of you isn't left waiting a lifetime if there are missed connections.

- Choose the "alpha-runner" to direct your way through the other runners in the race. If your goal is to simply finish, having a leader isn't crucial, but if you have even one eye on the clock, it's best to have someone be in charge of steering a path. Maybe even coordinate hand signals that mean things like, "let's pass this guy" or "I'm going full throttle."

- If you're a fastinista, consider wearing the same outfit or tops. That way, if you get separated, the lead runner can tell cheering bystanders to look for your twin and cheer her on. Plus, being matchy makes for fun race photos.

DURING THE RACE

9 Be honest about how you are feeling. If you're dragging, speak up. If you're raring to speed up, let your pal know. Staying silent only builds resentment, which you don't need to carry on your back in a race.

9 Don't run ahead and trot back (or, worse yet, run backward) unless your friend has signed an affidavit in advance that she's cool with that. Dimity's husband did the speed-up, slow-down thing in a half-marathon the couple did on, ironically enough, Valentine's Day. Let's just say there wasn't much love flowing from Dim to Grant race-day morning. (Dimity chimes in: Post-race, Grant told me he was "pacing me." Last I checked, a pacer stays with his runner, not 20 steps in front of her.)

9 Consult with each other before aid stations. "You need water?" or "I always walk when I eat my GU," are the types of communiqués you need to prevent losing each other in the shuffle. (Dimity, once more. Perhaps the only thing I didn't know about Sarah's running habits: She walks when she eats a gel. At a race we ran together, I impatiently encouraged her to stay strong and with me when she slowed to a walk. Little did I realize, she was simply refilling her tank. Got the memo now.)

POST-RACE

9 Meet at the agreed-upon location. (Now's the time for me to apologize, again, to Courtenay for not being able to find the media tent and hoofing it back to the hotel instead. So sorry, my friend!)

9 Chat about your race, whether you ran it together or separately. Obviously, be sensitive to your friend's feelings about her finish. Again, honesty is the best policy (oh, gosh, I'm turning into my mother, aren't I?): If you're feeling cruddy about your time, 'fess up, but don't have an extended pity party if your pal is celebrating.

9 Snap some pics together, whether or not you crossed the line as a team. You were there for each other in spirit, and a picture to prove it, as the cliché goes, is worth a thousand words.

The pace required to cover 13.1 miles is also a thing of beauty. Metaphorically speaking, the race doesn't require freeway-worthy speeds, like a 5K, or the school-zone ones better suited for a marathon. Instead, you're somewhere in the 35-MPH cruising zone. You're definitely moving, but you're not frantic from oxygen deprivation and continual muscle burn. (Or at least not until mile 10 or so.) Plus, the distance is long enough that you can make great gains in time by speeding up only slightly; a doable 15-second drop in your average pace nets a more than 3-minute improvement in your finishing time.

Come race day, a half-marathon makes you feel like a legit runner; at the bigger races, you may be running at the same time as elite runners, who finish a full marathon in the time it takes me to finish a half. (Disregard this fact.) Come to the starting line with both a race plan and the knowledge that the race is long and, at some point, you're just going to have to hang in there. Merely going out there and "seeing how it goes" makes for a long day. (Trust me on that one.) Like all races, a half-marathon is most efficiently run with the goal of either keeping even splits or running the first half slower than the second, which is—*say it with me*—a negative split. Unless I walk the first 2 miles, I have a very hard time running a negative split or staying with any race plan. In fact, despite what I have plotted out pre-race, most of my half-marathons end up looking something like this:

Mile 1: Get too carried away by the cheering crowds, who are lured by the word *marathon*. The average bystander may not know what a 10K is, but nearly everybody knows what a marathon is (even if they only know it in a TV context, à la *The Real Housewives of Orange County* marathon). So a half is a little shorter than a marathon. That's for them to figure out as I go out too fast.

Mile 2: Slow down, because mile 1 and 2 are, after all, my warm-up miles.

Mile 3 to 6.55: Check out my fellow racers, look for funny signs, generally feel good, and settle into a rhythm as I wait for the halfway point.

Mile 6.55: Halfway done! Wait, only halfway done? I still have to go as far as I just came?

Mile 7 to 11: Acknowledge a half-marathon is not an insignificant distance; my knees, my back, and my head support that notion. Despite unconsciously slowing down more than I'd like to, I do my best to hang tough, like New Kids on the Block taught me how to do, back when I hijacked my mom's Dodge Caravan radio.

Mile 11 to 13: Hang in there, hang in there, hang *in* there. Pick up the pace if I possess both the motivation and the energy reserves, but usually, one of the two, or both, is lacking.

Mile 13 to 13.1: Pick it up. For real. Cross the finish line and feel incredibly happy about two things: 1. the race is over, and 2. I ran a half-marathon!

The last reason I love the half-marathon? I'll be honest: Most likely I will never run another marathon. My body and my life are both more fragile than I'd like to admit. So when my running ego needs some distance glory, it has to come from the half-marathon. Not *just* the half-marathon. *The* half-marathon.

HALF-MARATHON: FINISH IT

"A half-marathon is perfect for a busy mama: long enough to get into the meat of training, but not so long that the baby needs to eat halfway into a training run."

—KATE

Best for: Runners who want to tackle the anthem race for mother runners: a beautifully odd 13.1 miles.

Physical Prereq: The ability to comfortably finish a 6-mile run is preferred, as is experience in some shorter races. (If you don't have the former, build up to it and throw in a race or two while you do so.)

Plan Overview: This plan, a little short of four months long, will comfortably bring you up to half-marathon glory. Most of the runs are at an easy pace, making it perfect for a pair or group of women to take it on together: lots and lots of time to talk. Working your long runs up to race distance gets you ready mentally and physically prepped for the half challenge, but a range is given in later weeks to accommodate all levels (or if it seems overwhelming). From the start, the plan integrates short bits of intensity and start-slow-get-faster race strategy, kind of like how you try to "hide" shredded zucchini in spaghetti sauce.

HALF-MARATHON: Finish It

Quick Key:

= Bail if necessary.

= Bailing is not an option.

CD = Cool down
E = Easy
H = Hills
I = Interval

LR = Long run
WU = Warm-up
XT = Crosstrain
Z = Zone (see page 118 for definitions)

WEEK	MONDAY	TUESDAY	WEDNESDAY	THURSDAY	FRIDAY	SATURDAY	SUNDAY
1	[1]E: 3 miles + 4 strides; or XT[2]	E: 4–5 miles[3]	XT; or rest[4]	3–4 miles as 10 minute WU; I: 6 x 30 sec at Z4–5 w/1 min. recovery; 10 min CD[5]	E: 3 miles; or XT	[6]LR: 6 miles [7]	Rest[8]
2	Fun workout[9]	E: 5 miles	XT; or rest	E: 4 miles	E: 3 miles; or XT	LR: 7 miles	Rest
3	E: 3 miles + 4 strides; or XT	E: 6 miles	Rest	3 miles as 10 min WU; H: 4 x 45 sec in Z4–5; 10 min CD	E: 4 miles; or XT	LR: 8 miles	Rest
4	Fun workout	E: 7 miles	XT; or rest	3 miles as 10 min WU; I: 6 x 1 min. in Z4 w/2 min recovery; 10 min CD	E: 4 miles; or XT	LR: 7 miles	Rest
5	E: 3 miles + 6 strides; or XT	E: 5 miles	XT; or rest	E: 3–5 miles[10]	E: 3 miles; or XT	LR: 8 miles	Rest
6	E: 3 miles + 6 strides; or XT	E: 6 miles	Rest	3 miles as 10 min WU; H: 6 x 45 sec in Z4–5; 10 min CD	E: 3 miles; or XT	LR: 9 miles	Rest
7	Fun workout	E: 7 miles	XT; or rest	E: 5 miles	E: 4 miles; or XT	LR: 12 miles, 10 min. strong finish[11]	Rest

HALF-MARATHON: Finish It *continued*

8	E: 3 miles + 8 strides; or XT	E: 5 miles	XT; or rest	E: 4–6 miles	E: 3 miles; or XT	LR: 10 miles	Rest
9	E: 3 miles + 8 strides; or XT	E: 6 miles	Rest	3 miles as 10 min WU; H: 6 x 1 min. at Z4–5; 10 min CD	E: 4 miles; or XT	LR: 10–12 miles	Rest
10	Fun workout	E: 7 miles	XT; or rest	3–4 miles as 10 min WU; I: 8 x 1 min. in Z4–5 w/2 min recovery; 10 min CD	E: 3 miles; or XT	LR: 8 miles, 10 min. strong finish	Rest
11	E: 3 miles + 10 strides; or XT	E: 4 miles	E: 3 miles	E: 4–6 miles	XT; or rest	LR: 10 miles	Rest
12	E: 3 miles + 10 strides; or XT	E: 6 miles	Rest	E: 5–6 miles	E: 4 miles; or XT	LR: 11–13 miles	Rest
13	Fun workout	E: 4 miles	XT; or rest	3–4 miles as 10 min WU; I: 6 x 2 min. in Z 4 w/2 min. recovery; 10 min CD	E: 3 miles; or XT	LR: 8 miles	Rest
14	E: 3 miles + 6 strides; or XT	E: 3 miles	XT; or rest	E: 4 miles	E: 3 miles; or XT	LR: 6 miles	Rest
15	E: 3 miles + 6 strides; or XT	E: 3 miles, last 10 min. at RP	E: 2–3 miles	Rest	E: 30 min. + 3–4 strides	13.1![12]	Bling! Sport your medal all day.

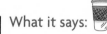

1 **What it says:**

What you do: If you need your usual running time to fill your empty fridge or take care of some other task, go for it.

More details: Once a week, we give you a get-out-of-jail-free card. No questions asked. Except maybe by your kids, who notice your low-endorphin mood: "Mom, why are you so crabby today?"

2 **What it says:** E: 3 miles + 4 strides; or XT

What you do: Pick your poison: a three-mile easy run, followed by four strides (short, steady pick-ups of pace); or a 30-60 minute crosstraining session. Whichever option you choose, keep it light to moderate in effort.

More details: To do a stride, find flat pavement or grass. Keeping your limbs relaxed, run as fast as you can for about 100 meters or 30 seconds. The idea is to teach your muscles to run fast without taxing your cardiovascular system too much. Take as much time as you need between strides.

3 **What it says:** E: 4-5 miles

What you do: Knock off 4 to 5 miles, preferably with a friend so you can catch up.

4 **What it says:** XT; or rest

What you do: Flip a coin. Heads: Hit the elliptical. Tails: Hit the pillow. (Or feel free to listen to your body.)

5 **What it says:** 3-4 miles as 10 minute WU; I: 6 x 30 sec at Z4-5 w/1 min. recovery; 10 min CD

What you do: Wake up your engine and legs for 10 minutes, then gun it as fast as you can for 30 seconds. Slow down significantly or walk for a minute; do six total of those suckers. Cool down your engine for 10 minutes. Expect to go between three and four miles.

More details: The mileage is simply a guide, so no need to run around your block one more time to reach three miles.

6 **What it says:**

What you do: Reschedule your week, hire a babysitter, get up at 5 A.M. Whatever you need to do to get this workout done.

More details: There's a weekly session that simply *must* be done in order to ensure success. There is, unlike what we do with our children on an almost hourly basis, no negotiating.

7 **What it says:** LR: 6-7 miles

What you do: Tick off six to seven miles.

More details: If you're dragging, aim for six. Motoring? You've got seven, friend.

8 What it says: Rest
What you do: Take the day off, or we'll throw some other (less gentle) four-letter words your way.

9 What it says: Fun workout
What you do: Turn to page 116, close your eyes, swipe your finger across the page, and see what fun you're in for today!

10 What it says: LR: 8 miles, 10 min. strong finish
What you do: At the end of your 8-mile run, pretend your kids are chasing you for 10 minutes.

11 What it says: 13.1!
What you do: No sleep till you've got a medal around your neck. Or should we say until your kid does? They always steal them, right?

TAKE IT *From* A MOTHER
WHAT WAS YOUR WORST RACE EXPERIENCE?

"Because I had been running for a few years, I (stupidly) followed an intermediate training plan for my first half-marathon. A few weeks into the plan, I dropped to an easier plan, but I'd already strained my muscles and never fully recovered. Race day was in the 80s by 9 A.M., and the 'downhill' course was actually 'rolling hills.' I was doing the zombie slog by mile 12, and it took me 2 weeks before I could walk normally again."
—LISA (Two days after that race, she played tennis with her husband. "Unless the ball landed within two steps of me, I just had to watch it bounce. I couldn't run for it.")

"Torrential rains, thunder, and lightning hit around mile 3 of the Providence Heart & Sole Women's 5-Miler. The water was up to our calves, but the adrenaline of the race kept us moving, and the threatening weather added to the excitement."
—BETSY (Favorite crosstraining event: swimming. "It's gentle on the body, cools you off, and who needs a shower after swimming in bleach?")

"I trained hard for the Chicago Marathon, but had an awful race. It was hot, and I puked twice afterward: once lying in a rose garden in Grant Park and again on Michigan Avenue in front of the Art Institute."

—EMILY (Favors the 10K Groundhog Run in Kansas City, where she can run underground in the SubTropolis, an underground business complex, in the middle of winter.)

"I ran the Polar Dash 10K in St. Paul on January 1, 2011, in windchill well below the -15 degree air temperature. I started out too fast, got leg cramps, and had to walk. My face mask froze, so I couldn't wear it. Then my face froze. Yards before the finish, my lungs couldn't inhale any more cold air. As I went lightheaded and started seeing spots, my friend grabbed my hand, and ran me across the finish line."

—JOANN (An auspiciously timed Saturday morning run resulted in her starring as the unexpected lead of a college homecoming parade.)

"I was out of my league at an off-road triathlon. The mountain bike section was two loops at a ski area, up and down the steepest mountain trails I had ever ridden. I walked my bike up the mountain twice and managed to ride straight down without crashing. I walked 95 percent of the trail run. I didn't quit because I wasn't hurt, so there was no reason I couldn't finish. I couldn't stop crying at the finish. Although there was nothing fun about the race, I'm glad I finished. Plus, I finished ahead of the seven people who quit."

—KELLSEY (After reading *RLAM*, realized she was a real runner. "I'm doing it, no matter how short, slow, or crappy the run.")

"My most recent half-marathon. I finished in my slowest (nonpregnant) time ever, and felt sluggish the entire race. It was in the middle of too many races, too much training. I felt completely defeated, as if my best running days were over. Major overreaction."

—MONICA (Warning: Never shave your you-know-what area the day before a long run. "Chafing. Just sayin'.")

"I can't think of one."

—KATIE (Strangest thing she's seen on a run: a naked guy hosing off his side yard at 6 A.M.)

> *"I s@#t my way through the Magic Kingdom and the rest of the Disney parks. It was the worst run of my life, and not the experience Uncle Walt envisioned when he created the happiest place on earth."*
>
> —MELISSA (Has run in Egypt, Israel, and Kenya. "No, none of the Kenyans' talent rubbed off on me.")

HALF-MARATHON: OWN IT

> *"I had both sex and alcohol the night before a recent half-marathon, and I took 10 minutes off my previous best time. Clearly, it's a winning combination!"*
>
> —JULIA

Best for: Intermediate to advanced runners committed to blazing a path to a personal record.

Physical Prereq: Mother runners looking to test themselves across 13.1 miles should have an established base of consistent running for at least the past 6 months, and be able to complete an 8-mile run. It also helps to have been intimate with more demanding workouts, such as tempo runs or negative-split runs. Prior race experience is *muy* helpful, as well.

Plan Overview: This 13-week plan develops speed as it builds endurance. With its varied workouts, there's little risk of burnout of either your body or mind. A swift half-marathon calls for a yin-yang of patience and aggression, both of which you'll hone over the next 3-plus months.

1 What it says: E: 3 miles
What you do: Run 3 miles at a smile-on-your-face pace.

2 What it says:
What you do: Move heaven and earth (and your family, work deadlines, and social plans) to get this workout done.

More details: A personal-best half demands both endurance and the ability to hold race pace to the end, making long, tempo, and race-pace runs equally critical. Make sure you do at least one of each of these each week.

HALF-MARATHON: Own It

Quick Key:

= Bail if necessary.

= Bailing is not an option.

CD = Cooldown

E = Easy
H = Hills
I = Interval
LR = Long run
NS = Negative split

RP = Race pace (see page 105 to determine yours)
T = Tempo (see page 213 for definition)
WU = Warm-up
XT = Crosstrain
Z = Zone (see page 118 for definitions)

WEEK	MONDAY	TUESDAY	WEDNESDAY	THURSDAY	FRIDAY	SATURDAY	SUNDAY
1	E: 3 miles[1]	[2] 1 mile WU; T: 2 x 1 mile, .25-mile recovery; 1 mile CD[3]	Rest[4]	5 miles as 10 min. WU; I: 1, 2, 3, 2, 1 min. in Z4–5 w/2 min. recovery; 10 min. CD[5]	[6] E: 3 miles; or XT[7]	LR: 8 miles[8]	Rest
2	Fun workout[9]	1 mile WU; T: 2 miles; 1 mile CD	Rest	NS: 5 miles (3, 2)[10]	E: 3 miles; or XT	LR: 10 miles, mid 2 miles at RP[11]	Rest
3	E: 3 miles	1 mile WU; T: 3 x 1 mile w/ .25-mile recovery; 1 mile CD	Rest	5 miles as 10 min. WU; H: 6 x 1 min. in Z5; 10 min. CD[12]	E: 3 miles; or XT	LR: 12 miles, mid 4 miles at RP	Rest
4	E: 3 miles + 3 min. of 10 sec. in Z5, 20 sec. easy[13]	1 mile WU; T: 3 miles; 1 mile CD	Rest	6 miles as 10 min. WU; I: 4 x 4 min. in Z3–4 w/3 min. recovery; 10 min. CD	E: 3 miles; or XT	LR: 10 miles	Rest
5	Fun workout	E: 3–5 miles	Rest	6 miles, mid 4 miles at RP	E: 3 miles; or XT	LR: 13 miles, 10 min. strong finish[14]	Rest
6	E: 3–4 miles + 8 strides[15]	1 mile WU; T: 3 miles; 1 mile CD	Rest	NS: 6 miles (2, 2, 2)	E: 3 miles; or XT	LR: 14 miles, mid 5 at RP	Rest

HALF-MARATHON: Own It *continued*

7	E: 3–4 miles	1 mile WU; T: 4 x 1 mile w/ .25-mile recovery; 1 mile CD	Rest	5 miles as 10 min. WU; H: 6 x 2 min. in Z4–5; 10 min. CD	Fun workout	LR: 10 miles	Rest
8	E: 3–5 miles + 3 min. of 15 sec. in Z5, 15 sec. easy	1 mile WU; T: 2 x 2 mile w/ .25-mile recovery; 1 mile CD	Rest	5 miles as 10 min. WU; I: 2 x (1, 2, 3, 2, 1 min.) in Z4–5 w/2 min. recovery, and 5 min. recovery between sets; 10 min. CD	E: 3 miles; or XT	LR: 13 miles, 15 min. strong finish	Rest
9	E: 3–5 miles	1 mile WU; T: 4 miles; 1 mile CD	Rest	7 miles as 10 min. WU; H: 6 x 3 min. in Z4 w/2 min. recovery; 10 min. CD	E: 3 miles; or XT	LR: 15 miles, mid 6 at RP	Rest
10	E: 3–4 miles + 10 strides	E: 3–5 miles	Rest	6 miles NS (3, 3)	E: 3 miles; or XT	LR: 12 miles	Rest
11	Fun workout	1 mile WU; T: 5 miles; 1 mile CD	Rest	6–7 miles as 10 min. WU; I: 6 x 4 min. in Z4 w/2 min. recovery; 10 min. CD	E: 3 miles; or XT	LR: 10 miles, mid 4 at RP	Rest
12	E: 3 miles + 3 min. of 20 sec. in Z5, 10 sec. easy	4 miles, mid 2 miles at RP	Rest	4–5 miles as 10 min. WU; I: 5, 4, 3, 2, 1 in descending effort from Z3–Z4 w/2 min. recovery; 10 min. CD	E: 3 miles; or XT	LR: 8 miles, 10 min. strong finish	Rest
13	E: 3–4 miles	3 miles, last 2 miles at RP	Rest	E: 3 miles + 4–6 strides	E: 20 min.; or rest	13.1![16]	Massage anyone?

3 What it says: 1 mile WU; T: 2 x 1 mile, .25-mile recovery; 1 mile CD

What you do: Run 1 mile at an easy pace, then run tempo pace for a mile. Regain your breath for a quarter-mile, and do it again, then comfortably run home. Or to the end of your treadmill workout.

4 What it says: Rest

What you do: Be kind to your body and let it soak up your hard work and make you stronger.

5 What it says: 5 miles as 10 min. WU; I: 1, 2, 3, 2, 1 min. in Z4–5 w/2 min. recovery; 10 min. CD

What you do: Run roughly 5 miles total. Start out at an easy pace for 10 minutes. Then run 1 minute in Zone 4 to 5. Slow down for 2 minutes to recover, then hit Zone 4 to 5 for 2 minutes. Recover again for 2 minutes, then speed up for 3 minutes. Recover for 2 minutes, then zoom for 2 minutes. Recover for 2 minutes, then hit Zone 4 to 5 for 1 minute. (Phew!) Wrap up your workout with 10 easy minutes of running after the final 1-minute interval.

More details: This workout is called a ladder because you go up, then down in either time or distance. While it looks a trifle confusing on paper, trust us: You'll get into a rhythm sooner rather than later.

6 What it says:

What you do: We give you a pass to skip this workout if you want.

More details: Feel free to rearrange runs to ensure getting in the critical ones (see number 2), but don't run back-to-back harder sessions. Better to just skip one and be over-rested than overtrained.

7 What it says: E: 3 miles; or XT

What you do: Cruise for 3 miles, or opt to crosstrain.

8 What it says: LR: 8 miles

What you do: Cover 8 miles at a comfortable pace. Daydreaming about race day is optional.

9 What it says: Fun workout

What you do: Put the fun back in running by not running and heading to page 116 instead to pick a diversion to do today.

10 What it says: NS: 5 miles (3, 2)
What you do: Run for a total of 5 miles with each of the last 2 averaging a faster pace than each of the first 3.
More details: Running negative splits teaches your legs (and mind) how to push in the later stages of a race—key training for setting a PR.

11 What it says: LR: 10 miles, mid 2 miles at RP
What you do: Run for 10 miles total: 8 miles should be at a long, slow pace, but for 2 miles in the middle, rev up to race pace.
More details: You choose which 2 miles you want to turn on turbo boosters: miles 3 and 4; 4 and 5; 5 and 6; or even 6 and 7.

12 What it says: 5 miles as 10 min. WU; H: 6 x 1 min. in Z5; 10 min. CD
What you do: You're going to cover about 5 miles, first by running slowly for 10 minutes, and winding up near a hill. Ascend the hill for 1 minute, giving it all you've got, then jog (or walk) down, so you can attack the hill for a total of six times. Do an easy trot home for 10 minutes.
More details: Yes, you can do this bad boy on a treadmill. No need to settle for just one incline for the entire workout. Mix it up between 4 percent and 10 percent.

13 What it says: E: 3 miles + 3 min. of 10 sec. in Z5, 20 sec. easy
What you do: Run three easy-paced miles. Then, for 3 minutes total, alternate running as hard as you can for 10 seconds and running easy for 20 seconds.
More details: You'll end up doing ten fast-paced intervals because each fast-recover combo adds up to 30 seconds.

14 What it says: LR: 13 miles, 10 min. strong finish
What you do: Run for a total of 13 miles, the majority at a relaxed pace. For the final 10 minutes, however, get a little aggressive with the pace.
More details: No need to set any land-speed records: Just up your intensity a notch or two. (If nothing else, as you finish, it'll make your neighbors think you breezed the whole way at that speed!)

15 What it says: E: 3–4 miles + 8 strides
What you do: Run 3 to 4 miles at an easy pace, then run eight strides.
More details: Strides are short pickups that turn easy workouts into subtle speed builders. To do: Find a stretch of flat ground. Run nearly all out for 100 meters. Recover for roughly the same distance, then accelerate again. Repeat until you've completed the prescribed number of strides.

16 What it says: 13.1!
What you do: Pin on a number, position your family at important spots, and get your race on.
More details: Don't neglect warming up before the race. Yes, it's a longer distance, but if you plan to race it, don't rely on the first few miles as a warm-up. You need to have your body fully prepared before you cross the starting mat. A short, easy jog, some dynamic stretching, and some strides will have you off to your best start possible.

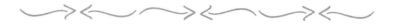

.1 AID STATIONS WE'D LIKE TO SEE
By Dimity + Sarah

Most aid stations are utilitarian: some water, some sports drink, maybe a gel or an orange slice if you're lucky. The best ones we've seen are at the Nike Women's Marathon, where you get a Ghirardelli chocolate (not really interested in eating it then, but good to save as a present for the kiddies); and at the Leadville Trail 100, where there's a veritable buffet of everything salty and sweet. But you have to go 100 miles to feast, which makes it slightly less appetizing.

This got us thinking about how we could spice up some aid stations. Note: Since we're in never-never land, it goes without saying that stopping at any of these would take no time off the race clock.

⚭ A make-your-own sign station, about 2 miles from the finish, where you could craft your own poster that said something along the lines of "Shut the f*&^ up! I'm not 'almost there'. But thank you for being out here."

⚭ A station with an espresso machine—and the guarantee that the java wouldn't erupt on you for the rest of the race.

9 A station with immaculate, scent-free, flushable Porta-Potties, which are magically cleaned and sanitized each time the doors are opened. Oh, and there would be actual sinks, too, with real soap and clean towels.

9 A station where Danny and Katherine Dreyer, cofounders of ChiRunning, would study your form, then make simple suggestions on how to get across the finish line with less effort.

9 A station that's the human equivalent of a car wash: You would pass through it on a conveyor belt as sweat, dried salt stains, pit odor, boogers, and leaked urine were cleaned off your body, hair, and outfit.

9 A station that knew what kind of music you liked and automatically downloaded a customized, brand-new, kick-buttocks playlist on your iPod as you ran by.

9 A station decked out with comfy chairs where hotties would remove your sweat-soaked socks; replace them with clean, soft ones; dump that pebble out of your shoe; and double knot your kicks with the perfect amount of tightness. Then they would give you a chivalrous hand to help you back up.

9 A station where, for a $50 donation to Susan B. Komen for the Cure, your kids would be guaranteed not to whine at you for the rest of the day.

9 A station where, for a $50 donation to Girls on the Run, you could buy yourself splits that are a minute faster.

9 A photo-booth station where you could stop in, get to see a previously taken shot of yourself in the race, then Photoshop it so it looks like you're blitzing along, with no thighs jiggling, no grimace on your face, no feet only millimeters off the ground, no muffin top inching out of your tank, no crotch bulge,[1] and no shirtless, potbellied dude sharing the frame with you.

9 A station a quarter-mile from the finish line where your running partner, lost in the crowd since mile 4, would miraculously materialize so you could cross the line together, hands clasped in triumph.

9 A station that, when you ran by, automatically removed all negative thoughts from your head. After you passed the table you immediately loved, loved, loved running; nothing hurt; you were totally meeting your goals; the weather was not too hot, cold, or windy, the course not too hard or hilly. Life is perfect.

---

[1] If, ahem, you didn't take our advice from *RLAM* and wear a running skirt or capris for race day.

06

THE MARATHON:
THE MOTHERLOAD

By Sarah

I have several versions of heaven. In one, after I enter the pearly gates, I immediately find out the answer to many of life's burning questions: What happened to Amelia Earhart? Who shot JFK? Who won the most votes in the 2000 presidential election? Is *American Idol* rigged?

In another iteration of the cloudy world above, I get to see all the times my path crossed with my now-husband while at college; we graduated the same year from Colgate, but we didn't meet until nearly 10 years later. He, of course, is constantly scheming to meet me, but I never notice him, à la a Cameron Diaz flick. (Hey: It's a fantasy; let me pretend I have flawless skin and a 36C rack.)

My latest spin on paradise? I get to travel back in time and run my first marathon after following a training plan. I figure if I could finish in 4:04 by adhering only to two loose training rules—to do increasingly long runs every weekend and to run a lot (maybe too much, in retrospect)—my mind reels at what I could have run if I actually would have put some forethought into it.[1]

A mix of naïveté and bravado prompted me to forgo a training plan—and any rest days. Some weeks I ran every day, others I got carried away with swimming and biking and hit the pavement only two, maybe three times. I did a single, solitary 3-hour run and hoped I covered 20 miles. (This was pre-Garmin, mind you—which now sounds about as primitive as "before indoor plumbing" or "the sports bra hadn't been invented yet.") God forbid I stretch, get a massage, or sit in an ice bath. And forget about taking in energy, like gels or chews, on the fly. I ate nothing, only taking in some sports drink. I also was clueless about ingesting a mix of protein and carbohydrates post-run.

---

[1] My seven marathon finish times clump around the 4:00 mark. My fastest, run in 2009, was 3:52, while my slowest, the hilly 2007 Nike Women's, was 4:11, with the 1999 NYC a close 4:10. Want to know my others? Sure you do, right? 3:59 (2010 Portland); 4:01 (2003 Napa Valley); and 4:01 (2010 Big Sur). At my debut marathon in San Francisco, I was young-ish (32) and had fresh legs; it was a perfect formula for a fast time, but I was ignorant of that fact. Sigh.

TAKE IT *From* A MOTHER
DO YOU WEAR YOUR GARMIN GPS ON RACE DAY?

"Yes, because I like to see my pace and splits. There's too much excitement to focus on feeling a pace, and I know the adrenaline at the beginning will cost me later in the race."

—CHRISTY (Group run funny moment: "I told someone I needed to go 'tie my shoe.' He proceeded to teach me how to secure a double knot. I had to explain what I really meant.")

"Not typically. Most races have the timers, and I don't need one more piece of equipment."

—EMILY (Shaved 16 minutes off her last half-marathon PR, despite 50-MPH wind gusts, downpours, mud, ice, and snow.)

"I normally wear my Garmin on race day, but I'm leaving it at home for my upcoming Olympic-distance triathlon. I'm going to trust my training."

—JACKIE (Influences her friends to race: "I love being side by side when gal pals complete their first races.")

"I have worn a Garmin on race day, but it doesn't seem to make a difference: 26.2 miles is still 26.2 miles."

—KATIE (Never squats to pee. "I pull my shorts and undies to the side, spread my legs, and let it go. Wearing a skirt makes the whole process a bit more discreet.")

"Yes. I like to know how I am doing at intermittent spots along the race, especially if it's long."

—NICKI (Her note to self: A close-to-50-year-old mother of six should not cough when running outside in cold temps.)

"No, but I've wanted to rip them off the wrists of runners next to me for their incessant beeping for 26.2 miles."

—TARA (Gets chills watching hordes of racers in front of her cross the starting line. "It's like a calm ocean wave.")

"I would lose my mind without my Garmin on race day."

—LORI (Cries every time she crosses a finish line.)

Fortunately, an Einstein's bagel was my daily breakfast back then, so by dumb luck I always had those carbs to fuel me. I had no idea how close I came to running sub-4:00 in my 26.2 debut.

Coulda, woulda, shoulda.

By winging it, not only did I most likely forgo a faster finishing time but also a better overall time: My makeshift training made that marathon a miserable experience. In the race, the 1998 San Francisco Marathon, I was hating life by mile 19—you might recall from our first book, I threw up flat Coke into my own hand—and was running on what felt like petrified tree trunks from mile 21 to the finish. I can still feel the immense, excruciating effort it took to bend my knees and lower my spent body to the grass in the finishers' area—and that was just a few minutes after collecting my medal. For days after the race, I avoided stairways like they were dark alleys and toilet seats as if they were covered in urine. Speaking of: My quads were so angry, a few times I peed standing up in my empty bathtub rather than squat on the potty. (No lie.) Let there be no doubt: My body wasn't ready for the intense pounding of covering 26.2 miles by foot.

Not only did I not train in a smart fashion, I had crossed very few starting lines of any distance. I would've been better off having a few more races under the waistband of my shorts. Before I toed the line of my debut marathon, I'd only participated in a handful of races, the highlight of which was the aforementioned 5K corporate fun run, where I almost beat my boss. Needless to say, I didn't stick to any training plans for those, either. Which sounds to me, a gal who now follows a training plan as closely as an engineer adheres to the blueprint of a suspension bridge, just like wearing blue lipstick and a buzzed haircut to an English Beat concert in my college days: crazy.

Race experience would have clued me in to things such as pacing (as in, don't expect to be able to run the first half of a marathon as speedily as you can complete a stand-alone 13.1-mile race); fueling (uh, maybe that Coke wasn't the best source of sugary carbohydrate to try to suck down); chafing (when not consumed with thoughts of my leadlike legs, I cringed at the rubbed-raw flesh between my thighs and under my bra straps); and dealing with pre-race jitters (hmmmm, maybe I would have been able to get more than about 75 minutes of shut-eye the night before).

Thankfully, I didn't let a painful experience ruin my relationship with the marathon. I've done six more, and I plan on running at least four more before I get my AARP card. I know quite a bit more now. Despite the math, a marathon is not merely a half-marathon times 2. I might have gotten a low grade in AP biology and not know the Krebs Cycle from a Krabby Patty, but even I realize something happens to your muscles, joints, and organs at an almost cellular level when you cover such a great distance.

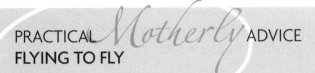

PRACTICAL *Motherly* ADVICE
FLYING TO FLY

Remember how safe it seemed to keep dating your high school boyfriend when you went off to the strange new world of college? The whole hometown-honey concept is applicable to running races, too. Whether you go cross-country or merely across a state line, it can be a bit overwhelming to contemplate an away race. There are a few things to consider before you register or head out of town:

TIME DIFFERENCE: If you're traveling west to east and arriving the day before the race, a 4:30 A.M. wake-up call will feel extra-brutally early. Consider building in a day before the race to acclimate to a variety of factors, including the race starting time. (And let's not forget your bowels need time to adjust to the morning ritual.) Another option: Start your acclimation at home. Incrementally bump up your waking and running time a few weeks before the race, so your body won't be quite so angry at you when you stand amid all the (peppy, energetic, local) people at the starting line.

WEATHER CONDITIONS: Temperature and humidity play a vital role in how you feel on race day. To wit: Dimity and I ran the Country Music Half Marathon in Nashville last May. Coming from Denver and Portland, respectively, Dimity wasn't prepped for humidity, and I wasn't ready for the humidity or the heat. When you're headed to warmer climes to race, do a few runs in an environment that comes as close to the race environment as possible. Run during the middle of the day, for instance, instead of the chilly morning, or run wearing tights and a long-sleeve shirt if you're taking on, say, the Honolulu Marathon. We don't recommend putting a treadmill in a sauna, but we've heard of it being done. Rest easy if you're going from hot to cooler temps; the chillier air is usually a guarantee of a good race.

ALTITUDE: Maybe only I waver on this consideration, but living at sea level makes me think long and hard about racing at elevation. When Denverite Dimity and I did the Ogden half-marathon, which starts at 5,000 feet in the Utah mountains, she enjoyed the net downhill course and ran like she was on her home turf—she basically was—whereas I was sucking serious wind within steps of the starting line.

Think about altitude as a factor like weather: It may slow you down, but it's not a given it will. Dimity has heard a handful of stories of sea-level women grabbing the Denver half-marathon by the *cojones*. The conventional wisdom is arriving the day before the race benefits you most, as your body doesn't really know what's going on; if you hang out in thin air for, say, four days, and then try to race, you might be caught in limbo land. Regardless of how your race goes, run by effort, not numbers; your 9-minute miles on flat land at 100-feet elevation might not translate so neatly to hilly miles at 4,000 feet. Finally, be sure to hydrate on the plane en route, before the race, during it, and post. Nothing kills the buzz of a race more than a dehydration headache.

SPECTATORS: If you plan to travel with your personal pep squad, skip this item. But if you travel solo or with girlfriends who are also going to be running, just remember there won't be anyone familiar cheering for you on the sidelines.

WHAT TO PACK: When you run a race in your own town, all your clothing options are at your fingertips. This is not the case when you're on the road, so you need to pack strategically and thoughtfully—or incur hundreds of dollars of baggage-check fees. Generally, you're good with two options for both your top and bottom, such as a long-sleeve top and a short-sleeve tee or tank; and either shorts or a skirt and capris or tights. However, you need oh so much more than clothes; check out our checklist on page 194.

PRE-RACE DINNER: Sure, it's a treat to not have to cook the night before a race, but eating in a restaurant means your options are more limited than they are at home. For bigger races or ones in small towns, search online for a restaurant months prior to the race and make reservations on the earlier side, as there will likely be a bunch of runners who need to be fed. Italian is always a good option, as are American-fare restaurants, where you can usually grab a salad and some form of pasta. I always opt for a salad and a relatively simple, noncreamy pasta dish.

MORNING-OF BREAKFAST: Searching a Monterey, California, supermarket for satisfying, make-in-the-hotel-during-predawn-hours breakfast options was honestly what made me opt to run my hometown marathon. It's tough for me to run 26.2 miles on an energy bar, a banana, and an Odwalla smoothie. Bring something from home, or stock your hotel minifridge. Yogurt with granola or a packet of Justin's Nut Butter slathered on a bagel satisfies, whereas I've found oatmeal made with coffee-machine hot water disappoints. Ask your hotel if it is laying out breakfast early for racers—and make sure it's going to be more than just coffee, juice, and stale cheese Danishes.

UNFAMILIARITY WITH THE COURSE: While I don't go so far as my pal Lindsey, who drove the entire 26.2 miles of Highway 1 that the Big Sur International Marathon covered, I do study a course profile like an eager 16-year-old with a driver's ed manual. I want to know where hills will greet (and taunt) me, and how many turns a course has. Dimity, on the other hand, pretends to study it, but nothing really soaks in; she ends up winging it. The beauty of her strategy? You don't have to fret about it, pre-race. You're at the bottom of a killer hill, and you have to get over it one way or another to see the finish line.

I'm also familiar with optimal training for me. It took me a few 26.2s, but I finally understand how to get across the finish line with a great time *and* attitude. Because I always have one eye on my finish time, I incorporate speedwork into my training, instead of forever plodding along at the same pace. This means I head to the track on Tuesdays and do tempo runs on Thursdays (if for no other reason than I like the repetition of all those "T" words. Track. Tuesdays. Tempo. Thursdays.). These specific workouts, complete with time goals firmly in mind, teach my feet how to fly faster and boost my cardiovascular fitness higher. Paula, my coach for my fourth marathon, once remarked, "An ugly duckling doesn't suddenly morph into a beautiful swan on race day." Translation: No matter how much you wish for it—like I did in marathons 1, 2, and 3—you don't magically become faster unless you occasionally train at a speedier pace.

Gone are the days of a single 20ish mile run: Now my plans always include three 20s, if not two 20-milers and one 20-plus. And, like all my runs exceeding 75 or 90 minutes, they include regular doses of energy gels to give me a boost along the way. (Amazing how that works.) These long efforts teach my body how to process stored fuel to sustain my energy level, and they prepare my joints and muscles for the pounding they'll take as I go 26.2.

Compared with the ignorance of my youth, when I was sure more was better, I also now religiously take a weekly rest day. This day off, with no crosstraining or even much walking (yes, I consciously limit my exertion as much as a mama of three can), allows my body to synthesize all the lessons I've taught it in the past week and emerge stronger. Sure, I'd be lying if I said rest days are mentally easy for me. Once a borderline exercise addict, always one. But the more I realize the benefits, such as renewed energy and lower split times, the easier it becomes.

With these cornerstones in place, I love marathon training. Honestly: L-O-V-E. Rarely do I feel more focused, yet at ease, in my running. There's no waffling about how long or hard to run. The answer is spelled out for me in black and white on a weekly schedule. Few things beat the sense of accomplishment I feel every day when I know I've run the distance or speed required to carry me across the finish line of my chosen 'thon. As a mom, there's rarely a chance to place a checkmark in a "done" box (there's *always* more laundry to wash/dry/fold/put away, right?), but when I'm training for a marathon, I get that checked-off feeling daily.

Plus, there's something wonderfully life encompassing about training for a 26.2-mile race; going to bed at 9:30 instead of sending out more e-mails to drum up auction items for the school fundraiser feels like an imperative, not a luxury. I'm forced to give some thought to what I eat for lunch every day instead of simply shoveling leftovers into my piehole. And then there's the perverse joy of subtly working in references to marathon training in daily life, say, at the post office or while waiting outside my first-graders' classrooms at the end of the school day.

PRACTICAL *Motherly* ADVICE
THE BEST OF TIMES, THE WORST OF TIMES:
WHEN TO SIGN ON FOR A MARATHON

My dad is an idiomatic southerner, quick to dispense advice, such as, "Let your avocation be your vocation," and "Don't make too many changes at once." If he were a runner, he'd add to the list, "There's never an ideal time to commit to a marathon." That said, there are certainly times in a busy woman's life that are better than others. Our take on them:

SITUATION: Trying to get pregnant

26.2? No.

WHY? You don't want to see that double blue line the morning after your second 20-mile training run. We applaud women who run 26.2 miles with a baby on board, but it's a tough road to hoe. Opt for shorter races.

SITUATION: Preschool kids

26.2? Yes.

WHY? You'd think older is better, but we found training with toddlers was less of an ordeal than we expected (e.g., we could take a joint afternoon nap, and we could have control of their social calendars). Now, with kids in elementary school, our weekends are chockablock full with soccer games, slumber parties, and art classes, commitments that seem out of our control—and that often conflict with the block of time we need for a weekly long run.

SITUATION: New job for you or hubs

26.2? No.

WHY? It's one thing to have your lunchtime run go long when your boss has witnessed your diligence for 6 years, but when it's the third week on the job, not so much. Plus, the stress of learning the ropes as you recover from 16-mile training runs isn't exactly ideal for your body. As for your husband's new gig: Give him the leeway to say yes to business trips or additional shifts without conflicting with your training.

SITUATION: New town

26.2? Heck, yeah (after you've unpacked the moving boxes and found your heart rate monitor and lightweight rain jacket).

WHY? You can explore your new environs on foot and hopefully make some running buddies along the way. Plus, you're going to have to stop in to your new local running store a couple times for new kicks; getting a relationship going with somebody who knows your feet and running habits is definitely a good call.

SITUATION: Banner birthday

26.2? Great idea.

WHY? Your commitment level will be higher if you're running to celebrate your 40th birthday. You'll feel you have more on the line, especially if you opt for a destination marathon and have some gal pals join you. Just don't be too hard on your not-as-resilient body if it decides to not cooperate and throws an injury your way.

SITUATION: Weight-loss quest

26.2? Iffy proposition.

WHY? While we firmly believe running is a great tool in the battle of the bulge, training to run 26.2 miles can result in added weight, not dropped pounds. You're ravenous during most of the training, and you've got 8 miles to do at midday tomorrow, so it's easier to justify a chocolate chip cookie as big as a Frisbee for a 4 P.M. snack. Yes, the weight you put on is most likely svelte muscle—and, as we've all been told too many times, muscle weighs more than fat—but if your emotional highs (and lows) ride on the number on the scale, it's best to stick to shorter races.

SITUATION: Fresh off an injury

26.2? Not a good idea.

WHY? Yes, you'll be raring to go. But why risk overdoing it and returning to square one on the road to recovery? Instead, give yourself time to simply enjoy the fact that you can run, and jump into some shorter races, if you'd like, to get back into the scene.

Looked at from the glass-half-empty perspective, however, marathon training does consume you for multiple months. The do-this-workout-today guidelines can sometimes feel constraining, even burdensome. Start by kissing good-bye any weekend free time, if you ever had such a thing to begin with. When 3, 4, or even 5 hours of a Saturday morning are eaten up by a long run, it's kind of tough to justify to your husband that you're heading out to a concert or happy hour with your sister.

Yet when the chips are down (read: My 6-year-old twins are engaged in their version of a WWE smackdown, or there's a flotilla of bake-sale cupcakes to be frosted), I can flash back to that morning's 14-mile river loop or memories from previous marathons. I have subconsciously collected a select repertoire of bright, clear moments that replenish my tank when I'm flagging, either at home or on the run. They appear without any prompting, as if my brain knows intuitively what my body needs to fare forward.

Perhaps surprisingly, one of my shining playbacks occurred during that challenging San Francisco Marathon. The year I ran the race, the course climbed a successive series of hills on Haight Street. Even though I'd done most of my training in tabletop-flat Chicago, it was early enough in the race that my legs had ample juice to power me up the inclines. I swiveled my head in amazement as I passed cluster after cluster of runners. Looking to my left I spied an auburn-haired guy wearing glasses and a big, goofy grin; it took me a moment to realize he was yelling out my name as he waved his arms and bounced up and down. It was Joe, a longtime pal. He jumped into the marathon, dodging runners to accompany me on my climb. Ever ebullient, Joe kept me laughing the whole way. Then, as quickly as he joined me, he hopped back to the sidewalk to spectate.

The hurt was still ahead of me, but for the next few miles, I ran with a smile on my face.

THE MARATHON: FINISH IT

"Dare I say my favorite distance is the marathon after only finishing one? I had a great race, and I love the response I get when I tell people I ran a marathon."

—RACHEL

Best for: Injury-free runners with four-plus relatively clear months who are ready to check a 26.2-mile race off their bucket lists.

Physical Prereq: Before stepping up to this plan, mother runners should have logged at least 9 to 12 months of week-in, week-out running, along with some experience stepping up to a race starting line. You should be able to run 8 miles comfortably and have no current shin splints, IT band issues, or other maladies.

Plan Overview: We're not gonna lie: Training for a marathon is a big deal, but this plan makes the path to it seem manageable. (Sort of like how bagged salads make including a veggie at dinner doable.) Training to cover 26.2 miles requires commitment, especially for the weekly long runs. On this plan, you'll do seven runs that are 15 or more miles long, which hone your mental toughness as surely as your calf muscles. This 20-week plan provides ample time to build, adapt, and be prepped to complete the mother of all races.

THE MARATHON: Finish It

Quick Key:

= Bail if necessary.

= Bailing is not an option.

CD = Cooldown

E = Easy
I = Interval
LR = Long run
NS = Negative split
RP = Race pace (see page 105 to

determine yours)
T = Tempo (see page 213 for definition)
WU = Warm-up
XT = Crosstrain
Z = Zone (see page 118 for definitions)

WEEK	MONDAY	TUESDAY	WEDNESDAY	THURSDAY	FRIDAY	SATURDAY	SUNDAY
1	E: 3 miles + 4 strides[1]	E: 3 miles[2]	Rest; or XT[3]	[4] 1–2 mile WU; T: 1.5 miles; 1–2 mile CD[5]	Rest; or XT	LR: 8 miles[6]	Rest[7]
2	[8] E: 3 miles	4 miles, mid 2 at RP[9]	Rest; or XT	NS: 6 miles (3, 3)[10]	E: 4 miles	LR: 10 miles, 15 min. strong finish[11]	Rest
3	Fun workout[12]	E: 5 miles	Rest; or XT	1–2 mile WU; T: 2 miles; 1–2 mile CD	E: 4 miles	LR: 11 miles, mid 5 at RP	Rest
4	E: 3 miles	E: 5 miles	Rest; or XT	1 mile WU; T: 3 x 1 mile w/.5 mile recovery; 1 mile CD	E: 3 miles	LR: 12 miles, mid 6 at RP	Rest
5	E: 3 miles + 8 strides	5 miles: mid 3 at RP	Rest; or XT	NS: 6 miles (2, 2, 2)	E: 3 miles	LR: 11 miles	Rest
6	Fun workout	E: 6 miles	Rest; or XT	1 mile WU; T: 2 x 1.5 mile w/.5 mile recovery; 1 mile CD	E: 3 miles	LR: 13 miles, 20 min. strong finish	Rest
7	E: 3 miles + 8 strides	7 miles NS (3, 3, 1)	Rest; or XT	E: 6 miles	Rest; or XT	LR: 14 miles	Rest
8	E: 3 miles	E: 7 miles	Rest; or XT	6 miles as 10 min. WU; H: 6 x 45–60 sec. hills in Z4–5 w/ recovery as needed; 10 min. CD[13]	E: 3 miles	LR: 15 miles, mid 7 at RP	Rest

THE MARATHON: Finish It *continued*

9	E: 3 miles	E: 8 miles	Rest; or XT	1 mile WU; T: 3 miles; 1 mile CD	E: 3 miles	LR: 16 miles	Rest
10	Fun workout	5 miles w/ mid 3 at RP	Rest; or XT	NS: 7 miles (3, 3, 1)[14]	E: 2–3 miles	LR: 14 miles, 20 min. strong finish	Rest
11	E: 3 miles	E: 6 miles	Rest; or XT	1 mile WU; T: 4 x 1 mile w/.25 mile recovery; 1 mile CD	E: 3–4 miles	LR: 17 miles	Rest
12	E: 3 miles	8 miles NS (4, 4)	Rest; or XT	6 miles as 10 min. WU; I: 2 x 30 sec., 2 x 45 sec., 2 x 1 min., all in Z4–5 w/1 min. recovery or as needed; 10 min. CD	E: 3 miles	LR: 18 miles	Rest
13	E: 3 miles	E: 7 miles	Rest; or XT	1 mile WU; T: 2 x 2 miles w/.5 mile recovery; 1 mile CD	Rest; or XT	LR: 14 miles, last 8 at RP	Rest
14	E: 3 miles + 10 strides	8 miles: mid 4 at RP	Rest; or XT	6 miles as 10 min. WU; I: 6–8 x 1.5–2 min. hills in Z3–4 w/ recovery as needed; 10 min. CD	E: 4 miles	LR: 19 miles	Rest
15	E: 3 miles	Fun workout	Rest; or XT	1 mile WU; T: 4 miles; 1 mile CD	E: 4 miles	LR: 14 miles	Rest
16	E: 3 miles	NS: 9 miles (4, 4, 1)	Rest; or XT	E: 4–5 miles	E: 3 miles	LR: 20 miles	Rest
17	E: 3 miles	Fun workout	Rest; or XT	1 mile WU; T: 5 miles; 1 mile CD	Rest; or XT	LR: 16 miles, 10 min. strong finish	Rest

18	E: 3 miles + 8 strides	4 miles NS (2, 2)	Rest; or XT	6 miles as 20 min. WU; I: 8 x 1 min at Z4–5 w/2 min. recovery; 20 min. CD	E: 5 miles	LR: 12 miles, last 5 at RP	Rest
19	E: 3 miles	1 mile WU; T: 2 miles; 1 mile CD	Rest; or XT	E: 4 miles	E: 4 miles	LR: 8–10 miles	Rest
20	E: 3 miles + 6 strides	4 miles: mid 2 at RP	Rest; or XT	E: 2 miles or rest	E: 2 miles or rest	26.2![15]	Brag to any- and every- one!

THE MARATHON: Finish It *continued*

1 **What it says:** E: 3 miles + 4 strides
What you do: A 3-mile cruise-it run followed by four short bursts of speed.
More details: Strides 101: Find a stretch of flat ground, either road or grass. Accelerate for about 100 meters or 30 seconds, then recover (slow down significantly, but keep moving) for about the same amount of time. Each 100-meter sprint = one stride.

2 **What it says:** E: 3 miles
What you do: Same as above, minus the speed burners at the end.

3 **What it says:** Rest; or XT
What you do: Take a day off—well, from exercise anyway—or crosstrain.
More details: Following a marathon training plan is a major commitment that can sometimes make even the most dedicated runner feel a bit handcuffed. Unlock those cuffs, if need be.

4 **What it says:**
What you do: Hire a babysitter, borrow a jogging stroller, or cue up *Megamind*. In other words, do whatever it takes to ensure you get this workout done.
More details: Long runs are the linchpin in marathon training and sit at the pinnacle of the priority list. There's no easy way to accomplish this other than by putting time on your legs. Second on the priority list are tempo and race-pace runs.

5 **What it says:** 1–2 mile WU; T: 1.5 mile; 1–2 mile CD
What you do: Run at an easy pace for a mile or two, crank out a fast mile and a half, then head home at a comfortable pace.
More details: Maintaining tempo pace requires concentration and motivation. I—SBS—find fast-beat music crucial in revving me up, so Rihanna and Nelly are often my tempo-run companions. (Well, their songs are, at least.)

6 **What it says:** LR: 8 miles
What you do: Run 8 miles at a cool, calm, collected pace.

7 **What it says:** Rest
What you do: Lounge as much as you can. Don't use the extra time to pick up an extra shift or help a friend move.

8 **What it says:**
What you do: Rest (or lightly crosstrain) if your body is telling you it needs a break.
More details: Easy runs and crosstraining days are the best to bail on, but with long-distance training, you can't always plan an off day. "Listening to your body" takes on new meaning. There may be some days when skipping the prescribed workout is the best thing to do. Don't feel bad, and—we can't stress this enough—*do not* try to make up any missed runs. Just pick up where you are on the schedule.

9 **What it says:** 4 miles, mid 2 at RP
What you do: Run 4 miles with the middle 2 miles at the speed you're aiming to maintain in the big 26.2.

10 **What it says:** NS: 6 miles (3, 3)
What you do: Run 6 miles total, with the second 3 miles faster than the first 3.
More details: Negative splits don't require sprinting, just getting progressively faster. These types of runs are excellent race prep: In a perfect world—no global warming, no civil wars, no traffic jams—you'd run the second half of your marathon faster than the first 13.1.

11 **What it says:** LR: 10 miles, 15 min. strong finish
What you do: Run 10 miles, upping your speed in the last 15 minutes.

More details: No need to sprint, just step on the gas slightly. When you intentionally finish a run strong, it helps in the pursuit of that elusive negative-split race (see number 10).

12
What it says: Fun workout
What you do: Kick up your heels at the pool, playground, or park.

13
What it says: 6 miles as 10 min. WU; H: 6 x 45–60 sec. hills in Z4–5 w/recovery as needed; 10 min. CD
What you do: Run for a total of 6 miles. Run at an easy pace, arriving at a hill (or incline on a treadmill) after 10 minutes. Dash up the incline for 45 to 60 seconds in Zone 4 to 5, followed by however much recovery you need (not *tooooo* much, though). Repeat the hill attack six times total, then cool down for 10 minutes.
More details: Intervals + hills = strong, eat-marathons-for-breakfast legs.

14
What it says: NS: 7 miles (3, 3, 1)
What you do: Run 7 miles, getting faster from miles 4 through 6, then crank it up even more for the final mile.

15
What it says: 26.2!
What you do: This is it, the big kahuna! Make us proud, mother runner, and show us what you're made of.
More details: Based on your long runs, you should have a rough estimate of what sort of pace you can hold for the marathon. It's smart to have a general idea for your first marathon, but keep in mind that finishing the thing is the main goal. Start slower than you think you should, maintain during the middle miles, and do what you have to do, minus jumping on your kid's back for a ride, near the end to make it across the line. As you reel in the last .2, tears in your eyes are optional, but pride is not.

TAKE IT *From* A MOTHER
WHAT WAS YOUR WORST NIGHT BEFORE A RACE?

*"I fell asleep after 2 A.M. the night before Ironman Wisconsin
and was awake at 3:30 A.M. for a nearly 17-hour race. But I didn't
falter during the race: just went slow and steady."*
—MARCI (Counts training for her first marathon with her fiancé as premarital counseling.)

*"The night before my first marathon, I was up with a feverish,
puking 18-month-old for hours. My husband tried to help, but
my son only wanted me. Somehow, I still did okay."*
—ELIZABETH (Strangest thing she's seen on a run: the tail of a baby lamb fly off while it was
wagging it. "I realize they had bands on to make them do so, but it really surprised me.")

*"I don't sleep well the night before any big race, but that doesn't worry
me unless the few days before were also bad. The worst was before a half-
marathon last spring. The week before the race, I caught a horrible cold
from my kids. None of us slept well the whole week, and I was grumpy
and anxious. In the end, I still set a PR, but I wonder how much better I
would have done with my good health and sleep routine intact."*
—TERZAH (Adheres to the superstition that you shouldn't wear the race shirt
in the race itself. "I like the idea that you have to earn the shirt.")

*"Definitely the night before I ran Boston, when I had flown in from
Russia four nights before and was sleeping on the couch at my parents'
house. My 11-month-old daughter was sleeping in the
Pack 'n Play inches from my face, and she woke up every hour."*
—HEATHER (Her proudest running moment: standing at the Boston Marathon starting line,
then running by the same hospital where she gave birth to her insomniac daughter.)

*"That would be the stomach flu 10K, with a 9-week-old baby nursing
every 2 to 3 hours, and my body trying desperately to empty
everything possible (from both ends) for two full days, including
the night before the race, which, of course, I still ran."*
—CATEY (Mother to three girls and five boys, ages 12 and under.)

> *"Getting home past midnight after spending the evening listening to hundreds of men in camo talk about guns and duck blinds at a Ducks Unlimited dinner with my husband. The things we do for love."*
>
> —HEATHER (Proudest running moment: when she realized she was running every day even though she wasn't training for anything.)

> *"I am not a morning person, so before every race I sleep like crap because I keep waking up, afraid I am going to sleep through the alarm."*
>
> —KATRINA (Usually runs around 9 P.M.)

THE MARATHON: OWN IT

> *"I'm so proud of my finish time at the Lake Placid Marathon. It was my fastest time ever. I just ate up the rolling hills."*
>
> —DEB

Best for: Another mother runner who has at least one marathon under her shoes, has done speed-work in the past, and has pinned on a race number (for a range of race distances) fairly consistently during the past 2 years.

Physical Prereq: You should be able to rip off a 10-mile run without it being too much of a hiccup in your life or on your legs.

Plan Overview: This is a fairly serious, intense plan that can get you a BQ or a significant PR, and, with either, some heart-swelling satisfaction. Over the course of 18 weeks, you'll be running four to five times a week, doing three 20-mile runs, and generally turning into a sleek, fine-tuned running machine.

THE MARATHON: Own It

Quick Key:

= Bail if necessary.

= Bailing is not an option.

CD = Cooldown

E = Easy
I = Interval
LR = Long run
NS = Negative split

RP = Race pace (see page 105 to determine yours)
T = Tempo (see page 213 for definition)
WU = Warm-up
XT = Crosstrain
Z = Zone (see page 118 for definitions)

WEEK	MONDAY	TUESDAY	WEDNESDAY	THURSDAY	FRIDAY	SATURDAY	SUNDAY
1	E: 4–5 miles[1]	1–2 mile WU; T: 2 x 1.5 mile w/ .25 mile recovery; 1–2 mile CD[2]	Rest; or XT[3]	5 to 6 miles as 10 min. WU; I: 2 x 2 min. in Z4, 2 x 4 min. in Z3, all with 2 min. recovery; 10 min. CD[4]	[5]E: 3–4 miles	[6]LR: 12 miles, 10 min. strong finish[7]	Rest[8]
2	E: 4–5 miles + 6 strides[9]	1–2 mile WU; T: 3 miles; 1–2 mile CD	Rest; or XT	7 hilly miles as 10 min. WU; I: 6 x 2:30 min. in Z4 w/ recovery as needed; 10 min. CD	E: 3–4 miles	LR: 14 miles	Rest
3	E: 4–5 miles	NS: 6 miles (3, 3)[10]	Rest; or XT	Fun workout[11]	E: 3–4 miles	LR: 15 miles, mid 5 at RP[12]	Rest
4	E: 4–5 miles	1–2 mile WU; T: 2 x 2 miles w/.25 mile recovery; 1–2 mile CD	Rest; or XT	E: 6–7 miles	E: 4 miles	LR: 13 miles, 15 min. strong finish	Rest
5	E: 4–5 miles + 8 strides	NS: 5 miles (2, 2, 1)[13]	Rest; or XT	7–8 hilly miles as 10 min. WU; I: 6 x 3:30 min. in Z3–4 w/ recovery as needed; 10 min. CD	E: 3–4 miles	LR: 16 miles, mid 6 miles at RP	Rest
6	E: 4–5 miles	1–2 miles WU; T: 4 miles; 1–2 miles CD	Rest; or XT	E: 8 miles	E: 3 miles	LR: 18 miles	Rest

THE MARATHON: Own It *continued*

7	Fun workout	NS: 10 miles (5, 5)	Rest; or XT	6 miles as 10 min. WU; I: 6 x 4 min. in Z3 w/3 min. recovery; 10 min. CD	E: 3 miles	LR: 20 miles	Rest
8	E: 3 miles	E: 7 miles	Rest; or XT	E: 8–10 miles	E: 3 miles	LR: 16 miles, mid 10 at RP	Rest
9	E: 4–5 miles + 10 strides	1–2 mile WU; T: 4 x 1 mile w/.25 mile recovery; 1–2 mile CD	Rest; or XT	7 miles as 10 min. WU; I: 8 x 4 min. in Z3 w/ 3 min. recovery; 10 min. CD	E: 4 miles	LR: 13 miles, 15 min. strong finish	Rest
10	E: 4–5 miles	NS: 4 miles (2, 2)	Rest; or XT	E: 5–6 miles	E: 3 miles	LR: 20 miles	Rest
11	E: 3 miles	1–2 mile WU; T: 5 miles; 1–2 mile CD	Rest; or XT	E: 7–8 miles	Fun workout	LR: 16 miles	Rest
12	E: 4–5 miles, include 6 x 10 sec. in Z5, 20 sec. easy[14]	8 miles as 10 min. WU; I: 10 x 4 min. in Z3 w/3 min. recovery; 10 min. CD	Rest; or XT	E: 7 miles	Rest	LR: 17 miles, mid 12 at RP	Rest
13	E: 4–5 miles	1–2 mile WU; T: 3 x 2 miles w/.25 mile recovery; 1–2 mile CD	Rest; or XT	E: 9 miles, last 4 at RP	E: 3–4 miles	LR: 15 miles, 20 min. strong finish	Rest
14	E: 4–5 miles, include 6 x 15 sec. Z5, 15 sec. easy	E: 8 miles, mid 6 at RP	Rest; or XT	Fun workout	E: 3 miles	LR: 20–21 miles	Rest
15	E: 3 miles	E: 5–6 miles	Rest; or XT	1–2 mile WU; T: 5–6 miles; 1–2 mile CD	E: 3–4 miles	LR: 15–17 miles, 15 min. strong finish	Rest
16	E: 4–5 miles, include 6 x 20 sec. in Z5, 10 sec. easy	E: 7 miles	Rest; or XT	E: 7–8 miles	E: 3–4 miles	LR: 14–16 miles	Rest

THE MARATHON: Own It *continued*						
17	Fun workout	1–2 mile WU; T: 3–4 miles; 1–2 mile CD	Rest; or XT	E: 6 miles + 4–6 strides	E: 3 miles	LR: 10–12 miles	Rest
18	E: 4 miles, last 2 at RP	E: 3 miles	Rest	E: 3 miles + 2–3 strides	Rest	26.2![15]	Avoid going down any stairs.

1 What it says: E: 4–5 miles
What you do: A 4- to 5-mile cruise.
More details: Keep it easy, grasshopper. You should feel energized and tank half full when you're done.

2 What it says: 1–2 mile WU; T: 2 x 1.5 mile w/.25 mile recovery; 1–2 mile CD
What you do: Warm up by running 1 to 2 miles. Run 1.5 miles at tempo pace, recover for a quarter-mile, then run another 1.5 miles at tempo. Slow your roll for 1 to 2 miles.
More details: Tempo should feel tough but not outer limits.

3 What it says: Rest; or XT
What you do: Rest or lightly crosstrain for 30 to 60 minutes.
More details: I—Dimity—would split the difference between resting and XT'ing and head to a gentler yoga class.

4 What it says: 5 to 6 miles as 10 min. WU; I: 2 x 2 min. in Z4; 2 x 4 min. in Z3, all with 2 min. recovery; 10 min. CD
What you do: Ten-minute warm-up. Run 2 minutes in Zone 4, recover for 2. Repeat once. Then run 4 minutes in Zone 3, recover for 2. Repeat once. Cool down for 10. Expect to go about 5 to 6 miles.

5 What it says:
What you do: If the universe is suddenly conspiring against you getting your run done, skip it—and don't sweat it.

6 What it says:
What you do: That workout, no matter what your week throws at you.

7 What it says: LR: 12 miles, 10 min. strong finish
What you do: A 12-mile-long run, with the last 10 minutes at a slightly faster pace. Aim for tempo if you can hack it. If not, just hang in there.

8 What it says: Rest
What you do: Rest.
More details: Don't make me repeat myself.

9 What it says: E: 4–5 miles + 6 strides
What you do: Run 4 to 5 miles easy, then do six strides: On a flat stretch of road or grass, pick up the pace to a controlled sprint—not an oxymoron—for about 100 meters or 30 seconds. Recover as needed between each stride.
More details: Strides aren't all out, but pretty close.

10 What it says: NS: 6 miles (3, 3)
What you do: Run 6 miles as a negative split, with the first 3 miles slower than the second half.
More details: It's less about how slow and (to some extent) how fast you go and more about not slowing during the last half of your run. Start at your usual easy pace for the first 3 miles, then slowly and gradually pick up the pace as you progress through the second half. Aim to go no faster than your marathon race pace. This isn't a speed workout, but a pacing workout. Picking it up even a little counts.

11 What it says: Fun workout
What you do: Flip to page 116 and spin the proverbial bottle.

12 What it says: LR: 15 miles, mid 5 at RP
What you do: A 15-miler, with five of the miles in the middle (miles 4 to 9, 5 to 10, 6 to 11, 7 to 12: your choice) at race pace.

13 What it says: NS: 5 miles (2, 2, 1)
What you do: Five miles, with the first 2 the slowest; the next 2, to borrow a word from my 5-year-old, the mediumest; the last 1, the fastest.

14 What it says: E: 4–5 miles, include 6 x 10 sec. in Z5, 20 sec. easy
What you do: Run 4 to 5 miles easy. Somewhere in the run, 'round about mile 3 or so, run 10 seconds hard (as fast as your legs can carry you), then 20 seconds easy. Crank it up a total of six times.

15 What it says: 26.2!
What to do: Run a marathon!
More details: Trust your training and race a smart race. One tactic Sarah has successfully used: Divide the race into chunks of 10 miles, 10 miles, and a 10K, and keep your brain focused only on the portion you are in. Keep up your fuel—remember you still need to eat and drink in the last 6 miles—and have at your 26.2 victory lap.

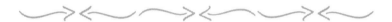

.1 FAMOUS WOMEN AND THEIR RACES
A group effort by Sarah, Dimity, intern Jessie,
and the Another Mother Runner tribe

When we selectively changed history in *Run Like a Mother*, we imagined what would've happened if famous women had been runners. This time we upped the challenge; now assuming that women all over the globe (and in the fictional world) are running, we wanted to know which races would suit some of them best.

ALICIA KEYS, with her empire state of mind, would stride through the New York City Marathon, while the streets made her feel brand new. "There's nothing you can't do, now you're in New York. . . ."

XENA would kick some ass in a Warrior Dash.

JOAN CRAWFORD, as we learned in *Mommie Dearest,* would certainly enjoy a Tough Mudder. Pretty sure her daughter, Christina, wouldn't be cheering her on from the sidelines.

THE GO-GO'S, that decidedly upbeat 1980s girl band with the keep-faring-forward name, would be the perfect candidates for a Ragnar Relay.

AUDREY HEPBURN would grace the Nike Women's Marathon for the Tiffany & Company finisher's necklace.

GLORIA STEINEM would revel in the female tribe vibe of an all-women's race like the ZOOMA series. For 13.1 miles, she'd carry a sign for her latest project. Anything for the cause.

BETTY WHITE would run the Leadville Trail 100, because that woman just keeps going and going and going.

MISS PIGGY would finally cement Kermit's love when she sets a course record for fastest swine at the Cincinnati Flying Pig Marathon.

JANE AUSTEN, JANE FONDA, JANE EYRE, JANE GOODALL, AND JANE LYNCH would all show up to do a See Jane Run race. JAYNE MANSFIELD, who rocked a nice rack, would get a special dispensation to join the crowd—along with a bulletproof sports bra.

WHISTLER'S MOTHER would rock Grandma's Marathon in Duluth.

KATE MIDDLETON was "to the manor born" to do the Disney Princess Half Marathon. She'd run with perfect posture and a dazzling grin, doing the docile royals' wave and never breaking her stride for the full 13.1 miles.

ELIZABETH TAYLOR would rock the Rock 'n' Roll Las Vegas Marathon; she could slip in a quickie divorce and marriage before the 4:00 P.M. start time.

SARAH PALIN AND MICHELE BACHMANN would train hard to qualify for the Boston Marathon, so they could be as close to the original Tea Party as possible.

SCARLETT O'HARA would have Mamie loosen up her corset so she could be gone with the wind at Atlanta's Peachtree Road Race 10K.

MARY-KATE AND ASHLEY OLSEN would star in Minnesota's Twin Cities Marathon. Although they'd be in their massive sunglasses that cover half their faces, they wouldn't wear matching outfits, so you could (kind of) tell them apart.

KATY PERRY would run the California International Marathon. In Daisy Dukes with a bikini on top, natch.

07

THE TOP TEN TRAINING-RELATED QUESTIONS[1]

By Dimity + Sarah[2]

1. HOW DO I DETERMINE RACE PACE?

An easier question might be, how do I create world peace—or at least peace and quiet in my household for more than 5 minutes at a time?

Seriously, race pace is both an art and a science. You can study pace charts and enter all your stats into online calculators for as long as it takes to run a marathon, and still, come race day, the numbers can mean nothing if your starting data was wrong.

The best race-time predictors are your previous races. By previous, we mean within the last year, barring any show-stopping injury or pregnancy. It's great that you ran a 3:32 marathon when you were 24. If you're 34 now, have had a kid, have been an off-and-on-again runner, and are aiming for marathon number 2, your time prediction isn't that lovely 3:32. But if you ran a 55-minute 10K six months ago, chances are, with some focused training, you could shave a couple minutes off of that time. That said, a 45-minute 10K probably isn't going to happen with only one training cycle.

A comprehensive online pace calculator that gives you mile splits for races, longer runs, speed workouts, and tempo runs is the McMillan Running Calculator (Google it), devised by noted running coach Greg McMillan. On the website, check a distance like 10K or half-marathon, type in your best recent race time at that designated distance, hit "calculate," and, voilà, up come predictions for every race distance and training-pace suggestions. (Race Pace, an SBS favorite, is a similar 99-cent iPhone app.)

---

[1]Beyond, how do I make it to the finish line?
[2]With serious input by Christine Hinton, the amazing running coach and ultrarunner who wrote all of the "Finish It" and "Own It" training plans in the previous sections. Just wanted you to know her expertise was still on board.

Bear in mind the numbers are predictions, not call-your-bookie sure things: Sarah's fastest recent half-marathon is 1:46:something. According to the McMillan calculator, she should be able to punch out a 3:44 marathon, which is 8 minutes faster than her bust-a-gut fastest 26.2. A 3:44 marathon is *not* gonna happen unless she hitches a ride for part of the route. Keep in mind that any race prediction, whether found in a book, magazine, or online, is for ideal conditions—as in your training has gone flawlessly, your body is humming, the weather is a cloudy and calm 55 degrees, the course is almost flat. Like we said, far from a sure thing.

If you haven't raced recently, another way to figure out proper race pace is to use Jeff Galloway's Magic Mile. In case you don't know, Galloway is the father of a wildly popular walk/run program, a training philosophy that includes short walk breaks at regular intervals. He devised the Magic Mile to help his athletes figure out their race paces, and he has generously allowed us to use it here. (It works even if you don't take walk breaks.)

1. Before you start any of the training programs in the previous chapters, run a mile. Ideally, you'd do it on a flat track—four times around is 1 mile—but if you can't swing that, measure out a mile on as flat a course as you can find.

2. Warm up for at least 10 minutes of easy running and walking. Finish the warm-up with four to six strides: about 30 seconds of focusing on quick cadence, strong arm swing, and acceleration.

3. Run your Magic Mile. Your pace should be challenging but not all out. Be sure to press stop on your watch when you finish the mile.

4. To get your current race pace—meaning, how fast you could run each mile during a race—do the following math:
   For a 5K: Add 33 seconds to your Magic Mile time.
   For a 10K: Convert your Magic Mile time to seconds and multiply by 1.15.
   For a half-marathon: Convert your Magic Mile time to seconds and multiply by 1.2.
   For a marathon: Convert your Magic Mile time to seconds and multiply by 1.3.

   Example: Say I magically ran a mile in 7:45.
   5K race pace: 7:45 + 33 seconds = 8:18 per mile
   10K race pace: 7:45 [465 seconds] x 1.15 = 535 seconds, or 8:55 per mile
   Half-marathon: 465 seconds x 1.2 = 558 seconds or 9:18 per mile
   Marathon: 465 seconds x 1.3 = 605 seconds or 10:05 per mile

5. Anytime you have "race pace" on a training plan, use your Magic Mile predictor, or a slightly more aggressive pace from a previous recent race. If you feel yourself getting faster and want to up the ante, do another Magic Mile and update your times. Don't go overboard, though: one Magic Mile every three weeks, max, please.

6. Take this with a huge grain of salt. Like all pace prediction charts, the Magic Mile is for racing nirvana, not Another Mother Runner reality. Instead, do your best to hit your paces while training, and then roll with the (hot, windy, sore-glute, period-started) punches on hard-training and race days.

2. CAN I MOVE WORKOUTS AROUND ON MY TRAINING PLANS?

Absolutely. If your long run needs to be on Wednesday, have at it. The most important tenet to heed when renovating is to stick to a pattern of easy/hard/easy/hard. Easy days are shorter runs with few, if any, accessories (no tempo, no speedwork, maybe a few strides), crosstraining days, and rest days. Hard days are the longest run of the week (regardless of pace), and any run with a pace or hill element to it. It's not bad to put 2 easy days back to back, but you're inviting injury (and burnout) if you do the same with 2 hard days.

Example: Here's the seventh week of the **10K: OWN IT** Training Plan

MONDAY	TUESDAY	WEDNESDAY	THURSDAY	FRIDAY	SATURDAY	SUNDAY
E: 3 miles; or XT [This is an easy day.]	4 miles as 10 min. WU; I: 5 x 2 min. in Z4 w/1 min. recovery; 10 min. CD [This is a hard day.]	E: 3 miles; or XT [Easy]	1–2 mile WU; T: 2 x 1 mile + RP: 1 x 1 mile, all w/400 recovery; 1–2 mile CD [Hard]	Rest; or XT [Easy]	LR: 8–9 miles [Hard]	Rest [Easy]

You could rearrange it like this:

MONDAY	TUESDAY	WEDNESDAY	THURSDAY	FRIDAY	SATURDAY	SUNDAY
1–2 mile WU; T: 2 x 1 mile + RP: 1 x 1 mile, all w/400 recovery; 1–2 mile CD [Hard]	Rest [Easy]	LR: 8–9 miles [Hard]	E: 3 miles; or XT [Easy]	E: 3 miles; or XT [Easy]	4 miles as 10 min. WU; I: 5 x 2 min. in Z4 w/1 min. recovery; 10 min. CD [Hard]	Rest; or XT [Easy]

TAKE IT *From* A MOTHER
WHAT'S YOUR FAVORITE WORKOUT?

"Eight-hundred-meter repeats. They're long enough to challenge me, but still short enough for me to feel speedy."

—LESLEY (In half-marathons and marathons, thinks of the last 2 to 3 miles as a totally separate race.)

"So far, 5 miles seems very comfy. I am able to run it while my oldest boy bikes beside me, and we talk the whole way."

—NIKKI (Must-have piece of gear: shoes, socks, really good bra. "Oh, that's three.")

"My short interval run. We have a 5K course around our compound in Saudi Arabia that is quite hilly. I combine hills and intervals for a killer workout that leaves me wrecked and delirious!"

—CARRIE (Gets her favorite workout done by 7 A.M., because it's 100 degrees by then.)

"I aim for 7.34 miles per run. I like the number 7, and I'm 34 years old—hence the number. After my birthday, I'll be running a minimum of 35 weekly miles and 7.35 miles daily."

—KAY (Caveat: Speed or terrain may vary according to energy level.)

"Still too new to have a favorite. I'd like to be able to run the 4-mile route near my house someday."

—ANGIE ("I've supported my husband as he ran marathons. Now it's my turn, and I've been running for 2 months. But in my mind, I've been a runner my whole life.")

"Mile repeats, increasing my speed by 15 seconds or so per mile. I do five to six of them and feel like a superhero the rest of the day. The first time I did that workout is the first time I really understood the runner's high!"

—KATE (Continues to marvel that she can be stronger and faster at age 39, after two kids, than she was before.)

"I love 10-milers, preferably on a fairly flat, crushed-gravel trail."

—ROBIN (Started running because her boyfriend's butt was smaller than hers.)

> *"My usual 3.5-mile course. It's simple, and there's not too much traffic."*
>
> —NINA (Considered herself a real runner when people started mentioning they saw her out running.)

> *"Five to 8 miles on a new trail."*
>
> —LESLEY (Worst night before a race: husband texted her at 4 A.M., saying he saw a lump/ tumor on their son's arm. No more sleep for her. At 7 A.M., he texted her again, saying it must have been the position he was sleeping in that caused the lump.)

3. WHAT IF I GET SICK? INJURED?

It depends on the severity of what's got you down. If you're out for a few days with a cold, simply pick up where you left off. There is no need to try and make up your lost miles, as you'll likely end up pushing yourself deeper into illness. A rule of thumb for sickness, BTW: If all your symptoms are above your neck—you have a cough, a runny nose, or a sore throat, say—you can still exercise if you're so inclined and not supine. If you have congestion in your chest, a fever, or massive stomach issues (like you're doing fartleks to get to the toilet), it's best to chill out until you feel better. If you have to take an antibiotic, tell your doctor you're a runner and you're training for a race.

For both sickness and injury, there is no magic number, such as 3 weeks, when if you're healthy again before you hit that mark, you're good to race, and if you don't hit it, you're not. Your ability to bounce back really depends on the level of fitness you had going in, the size of your speed bump, and your goal for the race. Regardless of where you were when you were sidelined, when you get back to it, expect to take at least a few days to get back to your old self. Cut your mileage in half and keep the pace easy peasy, or risk a relapse.

For injuries, there are no worries: Just keep running.

Kidding. Injuries are the same deal as illness. If you tweak your back and need to take 4 or 5 days off, don't fret it. Take care of it, crosstrain if you can without pain, and once it's feeling close to 100 percent, resume the plan.

If your shin splits are getting worse and worse and 10 days off of them hasn't helped, you might need to redesign your training and race plans. What that looks like depends on the severity of your injury—and the stubbornness of your personality. You may need to adjust your time goal from a PR to simply finishing. You may need to drop back from the marathon to the half-marathon distance. You may need to stop running completely and find a new, further-down-the-road race, which hurts to type and, I know, hurts even more to experience. Realize, though, if you run a race with severe pain, you won't just have to recover from the race, you'll likely have to recuperate from the injury, too. Then it becomes months, not weeks, off from our beloved running.

There will always be another race, but you have only one body for your entire life. Take care of it.

4. SHOULD I RUN OR RACE WHEN I'M PREGNANT?

The medical community—usually such an agreeable crowd (not!)—has yet to solidify advice for pregnant women who want to run. Some doctors are all in favor of pounding the pavement, while others tell perfectly healthy preggo women, who are already runners, to stop running. While no advice neatly fits one (belly band–wearing) mother, we think this advice from the American Congress of Obstetricians and Gynecologists is sound: "If you were a runner before you became pregnant, you often can keep running during pregnancy, although you may have to modify your routine. Talk to your doctor about whether running during pregnancy is safe for you." They also recommend you exercise or run at an intensity that allows you to talk. (It goes without saying, seek out a doctor who understands your lifestyle. She may not condone running, but you at least want her to get it.)

If running feels good while you're carrying your load and you have no complications, go for it. If it doesn't, know that not running during pregnancy won't make or break your post-childbirth performance. Keep moving, of course, but hiking, biking, working out on the elliptical, and swimming are all great options. Many new moms come back with a vengeance, thanks to time-strapped schedules that force them to run even when they don't feel like it and a newfound purpose (Me! Me! Me!). If you do pin a race number on your growing belly, keep your goal modest: to finish the race with both you and your piglet happy and healthy.

5. SHOULD I RACE BEFORE MY GOAL RACE?

Unless you're a brand-new runner, it's always a good idea to take your wheels out for a spin on a race-course. Not only does a race break up training, it also lets you figure out how your training is playing out.

TRAINING PLAN	SUGGESTED TRAINING RACES	WEEKS BEFORE GOAL RACE	STRATEGY FOR THE RACE
5K: Finish It	None		
5K: Own It	5K or shorter	3–5	Monitor fitness and training
10K: Finish It	5K	3–5	Develop race toughness
10K: Own It	5K or 8K	3–6	Practice negative splitting
Half-Marathon: Finish It	5K or 8K	4–8	Get used to the racing scene
Half-Marathon: Own It	5K, 8K, or 10K	4–8	Practice race-morning routine
Marathon: Finish It	10K	8–10	Develop confidence
Marathon: Own It	10K or half-marathon	6–8	Practice marathon race pace and fueling

Slide a race into the training plan on one of your longer run days that has roughly the same mileage you're supposed to go, and call it good. Your pace will naturally pick up during the race, when you're in a herd of runners. Any training miles you miss will be made up for with intensity.

6. WHICH RACE SHOULD I DO?

Wow, there are as many variables to consider as there are energy bars to choose from: distance, size, location, date, entry fee, finishers' swag, you name it.

Let's start with distance. A progression of distance is the most conservative approach to take: Start with a 5K, work your way up to a 10K, then go longer, if you want. You can dive into a 10K without doing a previous race, but we'd strongly recommend a half- or full marathon not be your first race. As much as we love these longer races (well, at least *one* of us loves 26.2s), they provide plenty of opportunities for the proverbial wheels to fall off the bus—not an enjoyable situation for anyone, but especially tough for a racing newbie. By starting off shorter, you gain confidence and savviness, along with endurance, which will all translate to longer races when the time comes.

Now, race location: Major marathons, such as New York, Chicago, and Marine Corps, are phenomenal experiences with crowd support you can only dream about at other races. But being surrounded by tens of thousands of racers doesn't make for fastest-ever times—instead, it makes for a ravelike atmosphere, so wear your party shoes and attitude. Some folks might find it tough to rev up the pace at a small race with no spectators, while others will value the minimal hassles at local races, such as easy parking, short Porta-Potty lines, and no backups at aid stations.

Finally, contemplate what other variables matter to you. If you're intent on sporting a finisher's necklace instead of a medal, look into a women's race; if you refuse to run in hot temps, don't opt for a summer event.

7. HOW MUCH TIME SHOULD I TAKE OFF BETWEEN RACES?

The easiest way to remember how long you should take to recover from any given race is to take the number of miles you raced—3 or 6 or 13 or 26—and take that many days either totally off or with easy runs (no long runs, no speedwork, no crazy hills). You can also check out our reverse taper advice on page 139, for more structure.

Once your legs feel like themselves again, you can think about your next race and your goals for it. (Well, okay, you can *think* while you recoup, but don't act.) If you're all about the social aspect of running—and the pre- and post-race scene—and you don't run especially hard on the course, you can enter weekend races to your heart's desire. If a race means pushing down the pedal with no letup until you see the table with bagels, you need to pick your races judiciously. (Or face the consequences of having your times flatten or slow or, worse, getting injured.) Also consider the impact racing has on your family: If it includes them, the more the merrier. But if racing is a mom-only venture, consider getting family—or at least significant other—buy-in before committing to a big race.

8. IS THE TREADMILL THE SAME AS RUNNING OUTSIDE?

Unfortunately, no. On the 'mill, there's no terrain variability, wind, or weather to contend with, and you've got a little belt under your feet aiding your effort. That said, the treadmill has its benefits: You can home in on a specific pace and hang there, and the little belt is softer on your joints than pavement or sidewalks.

Many people have done the majority—if not all—their training on a treadmill and subsequently torn up a racecourse, so don't despair if that's your only option. Keep in mind, hitting that speed indoors is easier than outdoors. To mimic the extra effort it takes to run outside, bump up the incline to between 1 and 2 percent. If you want more numbers, Google "hill runner" and "treadmill chart" to see how various inclines, from 0 to 10 percent, translate to different paces.

9. SHOULD I STRENGTH TRAIN WHEN I'M ON A TRAINING PLAN?

The rational answer: yes. The realistic answer: Squeeze it in if and when you can. A simple routine of body-weight squats, lunges, planks, sit-ups, and push-ups will go further, in terms of injury prevention and strength, than you think it will. There is a great routine in chapter 8 that you can do on a crosstraining day. Or tack on a few moves after your run: Even if you only do 20 push-ups and 40 squats twice a week, you're 40 push-ups and 80 squats stronger than you used to be.

10. ALL YOUR TRAINING PLANS END ON SATURDAY. WHAT IF MY RACE IS ON A SUNDAY?[1]

Go for an easy 20-minute trot on Saturday, if you're so inclined, then have at it on Sunday.

CROSSTRAINING 411

Crosstraining doesn't just refresh your spirit; it also gives your muscles a chance to break out of the rut running can put them in. Most of the training plans have a crosstraining day, and we encourage you to heed them. (Like we tell our kids: Do as I say, not as I do.) The guidelines set forth in our training plans should dictate the length and intensity of your workout, but the rest is up to you. Here are some—but by no means all—options that will enhance your running:

---

[1] Yup. Ending on an easy one.

TAKE IT *From* A MOTHER
WHAT WAS YOUR FIRST RACE?

"A 5K. One of the Stroller Strides instructors pressured us to enter.
I was intrigued and gave it a shot. That instructor moved, and I
became one, and now I plan on pressuring people, as well."

—MARIA ("I always run better in a group, even if I am the last one lagging behind.
I know I have to keep going. There's no temptation to stop.")

"My sister and I entered a Race for the Cure 5K in memory of our mom."

—JULIE (Lost her GU supply in the Porta-Potty at mile 5 of the Chicago
Marathon, and could not refuel until mile 18.)

"I entered an 8K in Richmond, Virginia, because my friends were
doing it, and I wanted to get away for a girls' weekend."

—MEGAN (Had always wanted to run and, at age 38, "finally didn't care
what other people thought as I huffed and puffed.")

"I entered a half-marathon because I never thought I could do it."

—NATALIE (Could not run to the end of her driveway when she decided to register for 13.1 miles.)

"My first race distance was 2.3 miles. Aside from the lady leading
it, I was the only adult running with 15 elementary kids."

—RANDI (Hates the stagnant air at the gym.)

"15K. I started running with my husband, and it was the first race for both of us."

—CHRISTINE (Used to be a cyclist, but switched to running: "The lack of equipment
needed was liberating, and the cardiovascular workout is superior.")

"I debuted at the Cherry Creek Sneak, a 5K, in 2008. It was my
first race since junior high. I rode that high for a week."

—MOLLY (Best recent race: Steamboat Half Marathon, fueled by pre-
race margaritas and quality time with her running buddies.)

Barre Classes You won't need to scrounge your daughter's tutu and leotard for this workout—a pair of running capris and a tank top will suffice—but these types of workouts borrow heavily from ballet and the Lotte Berk Method. The common theme is using low or no weights to do a high number of repetitions of exercises that are designed to sculpt elongated muscles. If you can't find a class in your area, check out a DVD and follow along.

Circuit Training This type of workout can be as structured or as spontaneous as you want. Head to the gym or work with what you have at home. Start on a cardio machine (elliptical, bike, climbing up and down a flight of stairs, jumping rope) for 5 to 10 minutes, move to a lower-body strength exercise (squats, lunges, hamstring curls, leg extensions) for a minute, move to an upper-body strength exercise (arm curls, pull-ups, triceps dips, push-ups) for a minute, and finally do a set of core strengthening moves (crunches, planks, bicycles) for a minute. Repeat the circuit (cardio, lower, upper, core) for the right-for-your-plan amount of time, finishing with an easy cardio cooldown.

Core Training Although it's nice to banish a midsection memento from pregnancy, the real reason for this workout is to exert and build up your core, the area from the bottom of your rib cage to the bottom of your glutes. Core strength is crucial to proper running form, as it keeps all the limbs in line, instead of letting them splay out like pickup sticks. It also improves your posture, which leads to enhanced breathing on the run. Don't just lie there and crunch: Options abound, from following a plan in a magazine article to doing a DVD workout to taking a core class at a gym.

Jumping Rope This is way harder than you remember it being in middle school, but the effort is well worth it: Jumping rope builds explosive power, which comes in handy on the hills and the last section of the race. Round up your kids for a jump rope or double Dutch contest. Whether solitary or *en familia*, it won't take long for your heart to get thumping fast. (Added bonus: Clenching your love muscles to keep from peeing yourself while jumping blows Kegels away.)

Kickboxing A kick-booty option, kickboxing moves your body across all planes of motion (side to side, front to back, diagonally). Going 3-D enhances underused muscles, evens out muscle strength, increases flexibility, and gets your heart and lungs working overtime. Most gyms offer classes, or you can easily track down a DVD at the library. If all else fails, box a few rounds on Wii Sport. Don't scoff: Coach Christine, an ultrarunning mom of two, was sore after a couple rounds.

Martial Arts From karate to tai chi, martial-arts movements teach patience, increase flexibility, and build strength and confidence—all skills that transfer neatly to running. Plus, you'll be able to defend yourself if someone threatens your spot in the Porta-Potty line at a race. Many dojos (martial-arts schools) offer free sessions before committing to a chunk of lessons.

Power Walking Most hardcore runners cringe when they hear a certain four-letter word—walk—but don't knock it until you try it for exercise. Keep your pace brisk and actively engage your leg and butt muscles. Walking increases your flexibility in the hip flexor area, a common tight spot for runners. Increase the challenge by walking uphill or at an incline on a treadmill, and seriously pumping your bent-to-90-degrees arms.

Rock Climbing If you are fortunate enough to have access to the great outdoors, find a group to show you the ropes, or stick to bouldering (navigating boulders as you stick closer to the ground, so no rope or harness is required). Indoor rock gyms are another option: Experienced climbers provide all the equipment and instruction, and you get a solid strength and agility workout.

Spinning Riding a bike to nowhere will get you to Destination: Fitness in no time. Take a class, or ride on the trainer solo at home. Pedaling at high cadence gets your fast-twitch muscles charged, whereas running focuses on endurance and slow-twitch muscle development. Occasionally kicking up the intensity, such as in a spin class, keeps the body guessing and adapting.

Swimming Nonimpact swimming allows you to escape the heat (or any other type of weather) while still giving your heart and lungs a decent workout. Up the intensity by throwing in some intervals or using some pool toys, such as a pull buoy (a Styrofoam doohickey you place between your upper thighs to help your lower body float while you use only your arms) or kickboard. Or dial it back in the other direction and Zen out with easy laps.

Tennis The side-to-side shuffling and running back and forth strengthens stabilizer muscles as well as run-specific muscles, and gets you winded plenty fast. If your serve isn't Wimbledon worthy, remember there's no line judge to dictate how you play; rallying is great exercise. In a pinch, do Sarah's childhood favorite: Hit against a backboard, cement wall, or garage door.

Yoga Like martial arts, there is a range of yoga styles, from superactive to one step up from a nap. Vinyasa is often called "runner's yoga" because the moves are done in a flowing style, leaving runners with a familiar "worked out" feeling. All forms of yoga improve balance, flexibility, and muscle control—qualities many runners lack. (Hey, you lookin' at me?)

Zumba Nothing gets you out of the straight and narrow mentality running promotes faster than some Latin tunes and a little rhumba. This dance-inspired workout is surprisingly hard, and who doesn't want to have a dancer's body? Don't take our word for it: Check out the transformation of *Dancing with the Stars* contestants.

FUN WORKOUTS 411

While we all love the one-foot-in-front-of-another activity, we occasionally need a break, even—or especially—when eyeing a starting line. Sprinkled throughout each training plan, there is the occasional directive to do a "fun workout." These are different than crosstraining: Yes, these workouts will elevate your heart rate but the aim is to give your mouth a workout as you smile and laugh. Take your pick—or feel free to think up your own.

AQUA AEROBICS: Jack (yes, SBS's 45-year-old man) insists the weekly water class he takes "is a challenging workout." We'll take his word for it, recommending it especially if you're looking to avoid impact.

BIKE RIDING: Don't go all Lance Armstrong on us; we're talking toodling around town with your kids, maybe hitting up the library and a snow cone stand.

CROSS-COUNTRY SKIING: It takes more skill than most other options, but if you know how—or are game to learn—strap on some skis, and make the best of a snow-covered landscape.

DANCE CLASS: Whether you hit up a hip-hop class at your gym or a Jazzercise session at the local rec center, you'll build agility, coordination, and fitness.

DODGEBALL: Believe it or not, leagues do exist. Bring back the happy (or painful) memories of childhood, while working some quick lateral movements and your upper body. Could be a good way to vent some frustrations, too.

FOURSQUARE: Okay, so you need three other players, but we love this recess-time standard. We don't have any proof, but play it vigilantly enough and we think it would develop your upper body and agility.

ICE SKATING: Whether at an indoor rink or on a frozen backyard pond, this is solid fun. Who cares if you end up cleaning up the ice with your backside?

INLINE SKATING (AKA "ROLLERBLADING"): Yes, skates with wheels still exist—and it's still a blast to bomb around a schoolyard blacktop or paved multiuse trail. Your glutes and quads won't soon forget the workout.

OBSTACLE COURSE: Draw "tires" on the driveway with chalk for some agility drills, use a hedgerow as a stand-in for the hurdles, and make a puddle a water hazard to be leapt across. You're only limited by your imagination—or until one of your kids gets hurt following you.

RELAY RACES: Take the kids to a park, or really go gonzo and enlist the whole neighborhood or first grade. Bring water balloons, eggs and spoons, potato sacks, and bungee cords (for the three-legged race, of course).

SHOOTING BASKETS: Play a spirited round of "horse" with your kiddies or maybe even an informal pickup game, channeling your inner Lisa Leslie.

SLEDDING: Enjoy the downhill—because the trek back up, pulling a sled loaded with a kid or two, will get you huffing and puffing.

SOCCER: Rally the kids or recruit some other parents standing on the sidelines while your grade-schoolers practice. Yes, it involves running, but it also develops coordination, something many runners lack.

WEIGHTED HULA HOOP: Hula hooping is, um, circling back into fashion, with classes offered in parks, at gyms, and on DVDs. You can find weighted ones, usually 1 to 5 pounds, at many sporting goods stores; they often come with instructions.

ZONE 411

Because you've got enough numbers in your life—height charts, your ATM PIN, the date of your last period, trying to figure out algebra and realizing that you're not smarter than a fifth grader—we distilled training speeds into five zones. They are based on a scale of perceived effort (PE), where 0 percent is lying in your warm bed and 100 percent is all-out sprinting because a foaming-at-the-mouth raccoon is hot on your heels. If you are a numbers gal, realize that these percentages don't equate exactly to your maximum heart rate, but they're pretty close.

ZONE	PERCEIVED EFFORT	GOOD FOR	TALK TEST	FEELS LIKE
1	60–70 percent	Really easy runs, warm-ups, cooldowns, and recovery between intervals or track repeats.	If you're running with a friend, you could just as easily be on the phone with her: You can chat about everything from babysitters to incontinence. Alas, you can't wipe down the kitchen counters, as you do when you're on the horn.	Trotting along, feeling fine. You could run forever. (Not really, but you know what we mean.)
2	65–75 percent	Easy and long runs. Top end tends to be about marathon race pace (except when you're gunning for a BQ).	The gossip run. Talk still flows as easily as Lindsay Lohan gets arrested for DUI; a Kardashian appears on the cover of *Us Weekly*; or pregnancy rumors fly about Kate Middleton.	A little faster than Zone 1 (Z1) but still comfortable. Good rhythm. You'll feel fatigued toward the end of longer runs.
3	75–85 percent	Tempo runs. Can equate to half-marathon race pace and, at the faster end, 10K pace.	Spotty exchange run. Not much more than "good job" or "how (gasp) much (gasp) longer?" coming from your lips.	A controlled and sustainable harder effort. By the last mile, you are definitely ready. to. be. done.
4	90–95 percent	Intervals, hill repeats, fartleks. A 5K pace tends to be anywhere from 85 percent up into this range.	All you can hear is heavy breathing and (hopefully) light footsteps. Grunting allowed, if you can muster it.	Slightly less uncomfortable than a root canal; more uncomfortable than getting a cavity filled, with no Novocain.
5	95–100 percent	Pickups: less than 60 seconds.	Nada. Nothing. No words. Just be happy that someone alongside of you is sharing the hurt.	You have to ask? Lungs, legs, arms, entire body are *en fuego*. (In a good way, of course.)

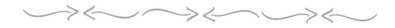

.1 FIFTY NEVER-FAIL MOTIVATIONAL SONGS
By Sarah + Dimity

While we agree that music has an amazing pump-us-up ability, we can't agree on the songs that get us moving no matter what state we're in when we hear them. Our solution? We each chose our top twenty-five inspirational tunes. (Caveat: We didn't repeat any songs in the three playlists in *Run Like a Mother*, thus the reason Springsteen's "The Rising" is missing from Dim's list, and Sarah left off Tina Turner's "The Best.")

SARAH'S GREATEST HITS

1 "Lose Yourself" by Eminem (Gotta lead with the obvious choice.)
2 "Fighter" by Christina Aguilera
3 "Crazy in Love" by Beyoncé ft. Jay-Z
4 "Moves Like Jagger" by Maroon 5 ft. Christina Aguilera
5 "#1" by Nelly (The title alone motivates!)
6 "Alive" by Pearl Jam
7 "You Shook Me All Night Long" by AC/DC
8 "Any Way You Want It" by Journey
9 "Runnin' Down a Dream" by Tom Petty
10 "Move Along" by the All-American Rejects
11 "Superman" by R.E.M. (If you can't tell, I'm into inspiring titles.)
12 "I Gotta Feeling" by The Black Eyed Peas
13 "Here Comes the Hotstepper" by Ini Kamoze
14 "My Body" by Young the Giant

15 "You Dropped a Bomb on Me" by the Gap Band (A psych-song from college rowing days.)
16 "Raise Your Glass" by P!nk
17 "Groove Is in the Heart" by Deee-Lite
18 "Here I Go Again" by Whitesnake (Mandatory fist pump; optional shaking of hair.)
19 "Heaven" by the Psychedelic Furs
20 "Eye of the Tiger" by Survivor (Pure cheese, but come on.)
21 "Basket Case" by Green Day
22 "Hard to Handle" by The Black Crowes
23 "Sense of Purpose" by Third World
24 "Gimme More" by Britney Spears (Gets me moving from the opening line, "It's Britney, b*#@h." Snarl.)
25 "More" by Usher (Give more, then even a little more. Empty that tank!)

DIMITY'S GREATEST HITS

1 "Walkin' on Sunshine" by Katrina & The Waves ("I feel alive, I feel the love, I feel the love that's really real.")

2 "Breathe" by Collective Soul

3 "Let It Will Be" by Madonna

4 "Closer to Fine" by Indigo Girls

5 "Slight Figure of Speech" by the Avett Brothers (A good beat and creative lyrics: two of my fave things.)

6 "Brighter than the Sun" by Colbie Caillat

7 "Little Bird" by Annie Lennox (Go tall women! Go little birds!)

8 "Bad Romance" by Lady Gaga

9 "Club Can't Handle Me" by Flo Rida ft. David Guetta

10 "Let the Rain" by Sara Bareilles

11 "Take a Chance on Me" by ABBA

12 "The Distance" by Cake

13 "Roll Away Your Stone" by Mumford & Sons

14 "Alex Chilton" by The Replacements

15 "Happy Girl" by Martina McBride (I always think of Amelia, my daughter, when this plays.)

16 "Good Things" by the BoDeans

17 "Accidentally in Love" by Counting Crows

18 "Praise You" by Fatboy Slim

19 "If You're Going through Hell (Before the Devil Even Knows)" by Rodney Atkins (Could be my race motto: "If you're going through hell, keep on going. Don't slow down.")

20 "Talk Me Down" by Gets the Girl

21 "Whip Smart" by Liz Phair

22 "Mary's Place" by Bruce Springsteen

23 "See These Bones" by Nada Surf

24 "Dog Days Are Over" by Florence + The Machine ("Run fast for your mother." Damn straight, Flo.)

25 "Don't Stop Believing" by the *Glee* cast (Yes, cheese, but I defy you to not sing along.)

08

STRENGTH TRAINING: PUMPING YOURSELF UP

By **Sarah**

I've never been a fan of lifting weights; I think it hearkens back to my introduction to the weight room during my freshman year of college. An eager novice rower, I set my alarm for the ungodly hour of 4:30 A.M., often mere hours after my head hit the pillow. Lifting weights was part of the rowing team's winter conditioning regimen, so insult was added to injury by the frigid, dark walk to the university gym during which one misstep could land a groggy student splayed in a snowbank. Huddled in the locker room, peeling off our heavy cotton sweats, my teammates and I would try to rouse ourselves by telling not terribly funny jokes, like the one that got the most laughs: "Time to make the doughnuts."

But no matter how much we warmed up, the weights were still heavy and the moves awkward for me. I still keenly feel the indignity of our tiny coxswain Kirsten, the gal who steered the boat, being able to lift as much—and sometimes more—than I could. Side by side on leg-press machines, she seemed easily to press 40 pounds more than I could; even on the cable row (the *row*!), the little cox could outshine me. It wasn't until a decade later that an exercise physiologist explained to me the reason. With my monkeylike long limbs, I had to push and pull the weights so much farther than compact Kirsten. Makes sense now, but at the time, I just felt dejected. And sore.

During the intervening years, I've flirted with weight training, especially after writing a "Defy Aging by Lifting Weights!" or "Get Fit and Firm at the Gym!" magazine article. I'll interview an exercise physiologist here, a kinesiologist there, and their expert advice echoes in my head. They make it sound so simple: A mere 20 to 30 minutes of lifting twice a week is all you need for stronger bones, more efficient metabolism, and a firmer butt. No three sets of 15 repetitions necessary, they assure me—one set of 10 to 12 reps will garner the same results. I mean, come on, how hard does that sound?

TAKE IT *From* A MOTHER
DO YOU STRENGTH TRAIN?

"Strength training gives my running more power. Plus, I am terrified of reinjury."

—AMANDA (Relies on ice, leg extensions, slower runs, and Advil three times a day to recover from knee pain.)

"Yes. My recovery and times are better when I strength train, but I hate doing it."

—CORRIE (Squeezes in 20 to 25 morning miles per week between part-time work, full-time school, and a house of three early risers.)

"I do now. After almost a year of injury, race, injury, race pattern, I've learned my lesson."

—ERICA (Best running moment: While tucking in her daughter, who was undergoing chemotherapy for a rare chronic kidney disease, Erica told her how proud she was of her. Her daughter replied, "I'm so proud of you, Mommy. Not everyone can run a marathon." "I do my best," Erica said, and then her sleepy little girl said, "Your best is perfect.")

"I was impressed by the results my friend was getting on the P90X program, but I wanted something free and not as structured, so I started my own Suck Less Challenge. A couple times a week, I did sets of exercises that would add up to 200 squats, 200 sit-ups, 100 push-ups, 150 triceps dips, and planks. For my first set, I could only do 17 sit-ups, 3 push-ups, 27 squats, 3 triceps dips, and a 15-second plank. After a few months, a typical night would look like this: 50 squats; 30-second plank; 50 sit-ups; 45-second plank; 25 push-ups; 30-second plank; 36 triceps dips; 45-second plank; repeat four times total."

—HEATHER (Has done this routine on the floor of the Atlanta airport: "Gross.")

"I haven't, but this year I've been going—and will try to continue to go— to a TRX class at my YMCA. Awesome core and strength workout."

—LOIS (Best thing she's heard at a marathon: a huge group of college boys yelling her name. "It was on my shirt. I gave them a fist pump, and they cheered even louder. It was right at mile 22, and it totally fired me up!")

"I do, but when my mileage gets up there, I tend to drop the weights first."

—LORI (Relies on tempo runs and hill repeats to improve her speed because intervals tend to injure her.)

"I should, but I don't really. Weights give me cement legs."

—NANCY (Favorite race: San Francisco's Bay to Breakers. "Everyone is so happy, it's a public party, and the course is beautiful.")

Tough, it turns out. The morning after an interview, I start with the best intentions. Because I'm loathe to give up a day of running, I run around our neighborhood for 20 minutes, ending at the gym. Lift for about 25 minutes, do 5 minutes of abdominal exercises, then jog the 5 minutes back to our digs. On paper it always looks so doable—and it is, physically. My main tripping point is thinking up a routine. Yes, I write about fitness for a living, but when I get to the gym, my mind undergoes the same transformation that hits me when I open iTunes or go to Barnes & Noble. Even though I can think of a dozen songs or books I want before I engage in the process, my mind goes as blank as an unplugged flat-screen TV the second I need to remember them.

Same thing happens when I walk into the weight room. I can barely remember the names of bicep curls and bench presses, let alone enough exercises to keep me productive for nearly half an hour. And forget recalling any tips about form. I only write the captions, I don't remember them. Because I favor free weights over machines—better because my body, not a contraption of metal, cables, and padding, is stabilizing me—looking at the little diagrams plastered to the lat pull-down gizmo isn't any help.

If there's a woman working with a trainer in the room, I shoot furtive glances at the duo, intent on stealing some expert moves. But I feel slimy mimicking the moves immediately, so I push out the few exercises my feeble brain can recall. Ten push-ups, 20 calf raises, and 5 minutes later, I try to act all casual, as if doing triceps kickbacks simultaneously with squats on a Bosu ball was all *my* idea. Yikes: coordination *and* balance required. I end up looking like a spaz in addition to a copycat.

So instead of knocking out a dozen moves, time drags and I lose interest. My best intentions to build bone and stave off the Grim Reaper wane, then months, and sometimes years, pass before I hold the heft of a dumbbell again.

This story could end with me breaking an osteoporosis-prone hip slipping on an icy sidewalk, but thankfully, I recently embraced group strength training, the perfect solution for me. No, another gal doesn't grab the other end of the barbell to help me hoist it—we all have to lift our own weights—but I love having an instructor dictate the exercises and watch my progress. I think of it as a personal trainer but way less spendy.

In January, I started going to a 5:30 A.M. kettlebell class. Even though I had to contend only with Portland's liquid snow to get there, the early hour had me flashing back to strength training sessions with the rowing team. The similarities didn't end there. Again, shorter women were outlifting me and I felt like a klutz. (If only my shoulder muscles were as well defined as my sports ego.) Within minutes of the first class, I realized I am utterly and completely devoid of any agility, coordination, or balance. I have endurance to burn, but none of the other traits that help define "physical fitness." Instead of focusing on the burn in both pairs of my cheeks, I entertain myself by trying to guess the instructor's themed playlists ("tunes about cars" or "songs about jilted lovers") and convince myself everyone else is working too hard to notice how hopelessly lame I am.

ENGAGE *Your* CORE LIKE THIS MOTHER
A PLEA FOR PILATES

By Dimity

Coming across the finish line of the 2011 Country Music half-marathon in Nashville last April, I looked down at my watch for the final time. My time was 2:02 and change, which was nearly 13 minutes slower than my half-marathon personal best—or, put another way, almost a minute slower per mile. So I wasn't exactly at my speediest. In addition, I was coming from Denver, my 5,280-foot-high hometown, and I thought the plunge closer to sea level would've mitigated the heat, humidity, and hills on the Nashville course. That wasn't to be: I was dehydrated, weary, and my head throbbed accordingly.

A wash of a race, right? Wrong. I was actually elated with every step of my 13.1-mile race. "I didn't hurt one bit," I told SBS, who finished several minutes ahead of me, as we gathered water and bagels at the finish line. "I can't even believe it. Not one step." Tears welled up behind my sunglasses as I spoke. For as long as I'd been a mom and carried my cinder-block children on my left hip, I'd had nearly crippling pain in my left hip and glute; the area was a tangle of triple-knotted nerves. The toxic web traveled down to my left knee and plunged a virtual railroad tie through my kneecap, and also migrated north to my back, which would go numb an hour into any longer run. Ibuprofen and just grinning and bearing it were my survival strategies, but they were far from solutions. Most days, I just wanted to chop off my left leg at the hip.

I tried chiropractic work (helped temporarily, but the bone-jacking effects would fade within 48 hours); physical therapy exercises (helped somewhat, but I was a slacker doing them); and finally, a doctor who ordered an MRI of my back. Diagnosis? Bulging L4 and L5 discs and arthritis commonly seen in a 60-year-old. "It's by far not the worst back I have seen," the doctor said, making me feel a little better, "but it's not in great shape for a 38-year-old."

I asked what he recommended. "Pilates," he said, with such assuredness I didn't have the courage to ask him for what I really wanted: cortisone or some other fix-it-all shot. I'd tried Pilates a couple of times, and to me it felt like an equipment-heavy, way-too-fastidious practice for dancers and their lithe bodies. I, like most endurance athletes, like my exercise heavy on sweat and endorphins. I like pushing myself harder and faster than I think I can go; seeing tangible, numeric results for my effort; and moving through the world powered by my two feet, not lying flat on my back in one place.

Trying to keep an open mind, I made an appointment with Marcia, a Pilates instructor whose path had crossed with mine. During the first lesson, we worked solely on the shush breath, a loud, strong exhale that shrink-wraps the entire torso and, when done correctly, engages the body so well it causes my legs to shake. I did probably fifty good breaths in a 55-minute session, and left her apartment feeling like I was already standing taller and stronger.

Slowly, over months of twice-a-week sessions—everything in Pilates is very mindful and sometimes, to my faster-is-better mind, painfully deliberate—I got the shush breath down, and we proceeded into advanced beginner moves, such as moving my legs while my core was engaged. The first few times, I couldn't lift my left one a millimeter. "Just visualize you're moving it," instructed Marcia. I eventually got that leg off the ground, as well as learned to balance my weight on both feet; got my hips back in alignment; and corrected my slump, a permanent fixture in my life since about age 9. I've progressed to the point where I can move my arms and legs at the same time, albeit only in wobbly sets of 10 that are more challenging than any race I've ever run.

At age 39, thanks in part to Pilates, I am stronger than I've ever been. I'm also slower than I've ever been, and, like a typical endurance athlete, that's tough for me to stomach some days. But then I remind myself that pain isn't ricocheting through my body with every step, and my runs aren't ending in my wishing for a new body, in tears, or in some combination thereof. And that result is worth all the time on the clock.

Emboldened, I signed up for boot camp, which involves demanding multimuscle moves (like chest presses on a stability ball as you bridge with your lower body) and provides more personal attention. I like feeling accountable to show up and perform—no cutting corners like I used to do when I lifted solo. (Okay, I may slack off just a bit when the instructor is helping someone else out and I just can't crunch my core anymore.) There are only ten of us, max, in camp, so there are plenty of opportunities for the instructor to correct my form and demand more of me. "Push that butt out and drop lower into that squat, Sarah," says Ashleigh, my instructor whose chiseled abs make it look like she lives in boot camp.

I'm now committed to these two classes: boot camp on Wednesday mornings and kettlebells on Fridays. I've been doing them only for 7 months, but already they are solidified as part of my routine. They splice up my running week perfectly: Monday I rest; Tuesday it's track or hill repeats; Wednesday weights; Thursday tempo; Friday weights again; Saturday long run; Sunday short run.

GET *Ripped* LIKE A MOTHER

We've all been there: trapped in the house with a sick child or napping baby, yet jonesing for a sweat session. Ashleigh Kayser, Sarah's booty-kicking boot camp instructor and mother of four, designed this 20ish-minute, no-equipment workout for situations just like these.

If you need a little side of cardio to go with your strength, turn this into a cardio circuit by inserting a minute or two of cardio exercise—running up and down the stairs, jumping rope, stepping up and down on a step, bouncing on a mini trampoline—in between each strength move.

TRICEPS DIPS: Position yourself in front of a bathtub or a low, sturdy table with your palms placed on it, fingers draped forward. Keep your backside as close as you can to the tub/table, knees as far away as you can sustain, with the ultimate goal of having your legs fully extended. Lower your body and bend your arms to a 90-degree angle, keeping your elbows close to your body.
DO: 15 reps, or what you can do in 1 minute.

STEP-UPS: Step your right foot up to a low chair or chest. Keep it on the top of the chair and raise your left leg up, leading with your knee. Then lower your left leg, and as soon as your foot touches the ground, raise it back up, leading with your knee. This is a continuous motion without any rests.
DO: 15 reps on each side, or 1 minute each side.

REACH CRUNCH: Lie flat on your back with your legs extended toward the ceiling and your feet directly above your hips. Raise your shoulder blades off the floor and reach toward your toes with your arms and hands extended upward. Lower and repeat. (Added challenge: Add a slight twist by reaching to the outside of each foot.)
DO: 20 reps or 1 minute, whichever is longer.

FROG JUMPS: Squat down, knees pointing slightly outward, and touch the ground. Using your athletic force, jump upward, bringing your hands above your head as though touching the sky. Land with soft knees and lower to the beginning position to repeat.

DO: 20 reps or 1 minute, whichever is longer.

PUSH-UPS ON A BENCH: Place your hands on a low bench or lower step. With your arms wide, your feet hip-width apart, and your spine, neck, and hips aligned in a straight line, do a push-up, almost touching the bench with your body. (If this is too tough, start on your knees. Too easy? Do the push-ups on the floor, or raise alternating legs for each push-up.)

DO: 15 to 20 reps.

SPLIT SQUAT: This move is part lunge, part squat. Stand with your back to any stairs and place your right leg behind you on the second step; extend your left leg in front of you in lunge position. Keeping your torso erect, bend your left knee until your thigh is almost parallel to the floor, keeping your abs engaged and your shoulder blades squeezed for posture. Make sure your left knee does not extend beyond the toe. (Hop your left foot out farther if needed.) Straighten the left leg and repeat. Switch legs.

DO: 15 reps each leg.

FLUTTERS: Lie facedown with your arms and legs extended straight, à la Superman flying. With your laces and palms facing the floor and your abs engaged, raise your legs and arms off the ground and flutter them quickly, as though you are a fluttering superwoman.

DO: For 1 minute.

SAILOR SIT-UP: Sit on the floor with your arms and legs pulled in toward your body. Roll back, extending your arms straight on either side of your head. Roll forward forcibly, placing your feet on the floor. Using core strength and momentum, rise to a standing position without using your hands, keeping your arms overhead. (Trust us: This is much harder than it sounds.) Hold a bottle of laundry detergent or a heavy can to help propel you forward and up if you are having a hard time getting off the ground.

DO: 12 reps.

ROTATION PLANK: Begin on your forearms and toes, with your elbows directly below your shoulders, and your neck, spine, and hips forming a straight line. Rotate your hips so they touch the ground on alternating sides without jutting your butt in the air. Keep your back fully supported and flat by consciously drawing in your abs.

DO: 15 each side (30 total).

HANDSTAND: Standing with your back to a wall, bend over until your hands are on the floor. With hands slightly more than shoulder width apart, crawl up the wall in one- to two-step increments until your feet are fully extended and you're inverted into a handstand. Stay for a slow count of five, then crawl down as quickly as you can. Repeat. (Wanna make it harder? Get into a handstand in one step and stay inverted for a minute. Or, harder still: Do an inverted push-up once you get up, working toward ten of them. And have a family member take video to send to us!)

DO: 10 times.

Thanks to group exercise, I've found both a bunch of great new songs for my running playlists and a host of exercises truly burned into my brain. You know how you won't ever have heard of a singer or a word, then once someone says it or you read it in a magazine, you spot it, like, three more times that week? Same goes for strength moves: One Wednesday in March, Ashleigh taught us a complex move called the Turkish Get-Up, where you start out lying on the ground holding a dumbbell straight up in the air, then perform a series of contortions until you are standing upright, with the weight still over your head in your outstretched hand. It was all Greek (Turkish?) to me . . . until kettlebell class just two days later, when one of the stations was, you guessed it: the Turkish Get-Up, with a light kettlebell standing in for a dumbbell.

The same thing happened with a tricky upper-body move that involved cupping a medicine ball in each hand with arms outstretched in front of the body, then opening up our arms toward the sides of our bodies, like hosts welcoming guests to our humble gym. It was a tough exercise, made harder by laughing through most of it when someone—okay, usually me—did Ricardo Montalban "Welcome to Fantasy Island!" impersonations. Then, there was the instructor this morning in kettlebells, showing us the identical move. (Such gracious instructors in Portland, I tell you.)

This morning's kettlebell workout also reminded me why I'm enjoying group training: Not only can I be a comedian, it also plays to my competitive side. (Oh yeah, you knew *that* was coming, right?) We had a substitute instructor, a hard-edged taskmaster who emanated an almost audible buzz even at that crack-of-dawn hour. She had us buddy up on a few moves, using our partners for anchors on stretchy bands and the like. Then she wanted to demo an abdominal move that involved Partner A throwing a medicine ball to Partner B, while B did sit-ups. The teacher scanned the room, fixing me in her sights as B to her A. The demo went on way too long, reminding me that *demo* is only one letter off from *demon*. But my ego, which is far stronger than my muscles, wouldn't let me crumble.

While no one has mistaken me yet for Jillian Michaels, my calves, arms, and upper back show more definition than they did last year. And running at race pace felt less challenging in my last two half-marathons. What's more, I'm having far fewer flashbacks to the collegiate weight room, which is a sure sign of progress.

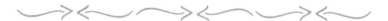

.1   THE COMMANDO WARS
By Dimity

As a community, we mother runners are fairly inclusive: You can be a country or a city mouse; a vegan or a carnivore; vote red or blue or Green; feed your baby your *leche* or formula; have a tattoo or not. As long as you like (or need) to run, you're in the tribe. The one sure thing to get people riled—or at least greatly entertained—is the subject of going commando, or not wearing underpants when you sweat. Despite both of us being avowed no-undies wearers, the tribe hasn't exactly fallen into line. Here, a sampling of answers to the controversial question *Do you go commando?*

YES	SOMETIMES	NO
"That's what liners are for." —ALANA	"I've been trying it out now that the weather is warming up. It's nice to have less for hungry cheeks to munch on." —CARYN	"I feel like my lady-bits are too close to the world, especially in the cold winter." —SUZANNE
"Digging for wedgies messes with my stride." —COREY	"Sometimes with the shorts that have the liner. I had terrible chafing with some cotton underwear after a half-marathon. I'll never make that mistake again." —JANE	"My running partner tries to convince me that it's better, but I think she's crazy." —CLAIRE
"I hate panty lines." —TERZAH	"Yes, in summer. In the winter, I wear ExOfficio undies because they are nice and toasty." —NANCY	"I tried it. I got blisters. No. Thank. You." —COURTNEY

YES	SOMETIMES	NO
"I wore underwear when I started running but realized it is much better to go without, especially on long runs. There is less chafing, less riding up, and no panty lines." —MELISSA	"I'm unaffiliated: Sometimes I do and sometimes I don't. (Honestly, it depends on what sort of, ahem, evening I had the night before. Blusssshiiiiing!)" —PHOEBE	"Nope. Never. But I have a special case (Mormon underwear) so . . . that's that." —ALISON
"Always. Don't need one more thing to worry about." —MELISSA	"Only with one pair of capris that I own, otherwise, no." —STACY	"I need to have the hoo-ha covered." —MICHELE
"I have undie-eating buns." —REBECCA	"Yes, in my skirts that have built-in shorts and shorts with liners. Not with capris." —RHONDA	"I am over 40 and have had two kids. I need underwear support." —ANDREA
"I can't stand pulling underwear out of my ass." —DARCY	"If the garment allows for it. I always wear a bra; though it's debatable if I need it." —SUSAN	"I have this irrational fear someone is going to pants me." —LORI
"Definitely, but I rely heavily on BodyGlide." —KRISTEN	"With my shorts and skirts, yes, but not with my compression tights. There's too much, um, drag." —JULIA	"I did it once, and my butt hurt for days." —LAUREN
"I hadn't thought of it until I read Run Like a Mother. I won't go back. It made me giggle at first when I was running, thinking about other people at the gym who might be doing the same thing." —SARAH	"I used to, but since having kids . . . not an option any longer." —CORRIE	"The seams on my capris/shorts/skirts all go up and down the center line and make their way into the tender nether regions." —TERRI
"I didn't used to, but after a run with a wedgie that wouldn't stop and some serious butt chafing, I will never wear underwear again." —AMANDA	"Depends on whether or not I have good underwear clean." —EMILY	"I wear yoga panties. They say you can't see them, but my 13-year-old always reminds me you can." —LAURA
"Swass [ass sweat] doesn't need an invitation to the running party." —TARA	"I have a $20 pair of Under Armour panties I wear when commando isn't appropriate. I think $20 for a single pair of underwear is ridiculous, but I'm a sucker. I paid it and I love them." —KATRINA	"I don't like feeling my middle belly jiggle when I run; sadly, my confidence increases if I have on some high-cut cotton briefs." —JULIE
"Hellz yeah." —CHRISTY	"Still trying to get used to it." —JOCELYN	"Ewwww." —KATIE

09

RECOVERY: ANOTHER MOTHER RUNNER SPA

By Sarah

Want to know what's in my bedside drawer? Let me give you a few hints. It's long and slender. It's hard in some spots, and flexible in others. Usually I use it on myself, but sometimes my husband does the honors. Either way, rubbing it on certain parts of my body makes me feel oh so good.

You guessed it: It's The Stick. (Wait, what were *you* thinking it was?)

A veritable magic wand for runners, The Stick is so simple, yet so effective. It has handles on both ends and hard plastic spindles covering a flexible bar. The spindles remind me of an abacus counter, except they are positioned evenly across the entire bar with no gaping space on one end. The 1-inch-long spindles can spin freely around the bar, but they can't move more than a millimeter or so from side to side. To use, an athlete grasps the handles and rubs The Stick back and forth across a sore calf or tight quad. Like many self-help tools, it massages soft tissue and releases fascia that's constraining muscles. Pressing down harder increases the effectiveness and ouch factor.

The first time I ever saw The Stick was in a van during the 197-mile Hood to Coast Relay. Amanda, one of my teammates in the Odyssey, dug it out of her gear bag after running a pretty-much-all-uphill section of the course. A hurt-so-good scowl spread across Amanda's face as she ironed The Stick up and down the length of her left thigh and outer hip. Equally intrigued and horrified, I asked her what she was doing. She said she swore by The Stick to release tension in her tight IT band. And she figured rubbing her quads post-run might prevent soreness and stiffness before running her final leg of the relay.

Hours later, as I watched Amanda triumph over the longest portion of the H2C after only getting fragmented sleep and ingesting fatty, salty snacks, I was a believer. Upon receiving mine

PRACTICAL *Motherly* ADVICE
HURTS SO GOOD

The idea behind most recovery tools is to attend to muscles and connective tissues before soreness can set in. But as we busy women know, sometimes our best intentions to roll and Stick is like making homemade tomato sauce: It just isn't happening. Whether you use these tools as preventive or after-the-fact measures, they'll serve you just as well as sauce from a jar does.

THE STICK: I've already familiarized you with The Stick, but I'd like to add that it is a 4-year-old ninja's dream play sword, so be sure to keep your new toy hidden.

TP THERAPY: Originally formulated by an athlete with fibromyalgia who experienced constant muscle pain and was told he could no longer exercise, Trigger Point Therapy is a series of at-home kits designed to mimic the benefits of a massage. While the specific area–targeted kits are a bit pricey, justify the purchase with the knowledge that it's about the same price of a professional massage. Used on key areas of the body to release tension and enhance blood flow, TP Therapy is your at-home masseur, no tip or appointment required.

FOAM ROLLER: Considered indispensible by many, the foam roller is an inexpensive (often less than $20) recovery tool. These rollers, available in smooth or nubby versions, take your at-home recovery a step further and attack muscle knots that can't be resolved by merely stretching. (You can even make your own foam roller following an instructional video on YouTube.)

TENNIS AND GOLF BALLS: Rolling tennis and golf balls under the foot helps to stretch fascia and ligaments in the foot, which can prevent foot pain after workouts and possibly plantar fasciitis down the road. We know many mother runners who keep a ball on the floor near their favorite TV-watching chair or under their desk at work.

DIY RECOVERY TOOLS

"A rolling pin. No joke. I even keep it under my side of the bed." —HEIDI

"I use my 4-year-old's XL super bouncy ball for my plantar fasciitis." —RACHEL

"I fill little Dixie cups with water and freeze them; they work great. I tear down the sides and can hold on to the cup while I massage." —TRACEY

"My 6-year-old loves karate chopping my legs after a long run!" —JENNIFER

in the mail, I rubbed it along my denim-clad thigh as I sat at my desk. Despite feeling perfectly fine pre-rub, my thigh muscles shrieked protestations, proclaiming tightness I didn't realize I had. I kept rubbing, and eventually the cries subsided, and it felt like healing juices were flowing across my (obviously) overworked muscles.

I wish I could say I started using The Stick as religiously as the pope says mass. But like Daphne, my younger daughter, does with a new Groovy Girls doll, I eventually lost interest and misplaced it. Months later, when I found it flecked with dust bunnies in a corner of my closet, I put it in my bedside drawer for safekeeping (and privacy, heh, heh). I broke it out last spring when plantar fasciitis grabbed ahold of my right foot and refused to let go.

Rub, rub, roll, roll. As I watched TiVo'd episodes of *Modern Family*, I massaged my overly tight calf, which my acupuncturist believed was contributing to my foot malady, and even endured the agony of using The Stick along my inflamed plantar fascia. While I was rubbing and rolling, 9-year-old Phoebe, my older daughter, walked through our room to get a drink of water. (Can I just interrupt my own anecdote to ask: Why do kids prefer using their parents' bathroom to the perfectly serviceable family bath?) She wanted to know what I was doing, then asked, "Can I rub your leg for you? Please?" I knew she was largely motivated by a desire to watch television, but I couldn't resist her offer. I sometimes lack the requisite masochistic streak to push hard and long enough to garner significant tension-relieving results, so I handed The Stick to her. From that evening on, my kids argued almost as much about who gets to roll "Mama's sore leg" as they do over playing with my iPhone. (Well, a chance to play Angry Birds trumps my rehabilitation, but still.)

Last summer, I also got Sticked by a pro. (Honestly, I didn't mean for that to come out as kinky sounding as it might seem.) I got to work out at E, a special part of Equinox gym near my parents' home in Connecticut, for research for a magazine article. Each one-on-one session with a trainer started and ended with a stretching session and Stick rubdown. The pressure was roughly ten times more intense than what my kids could serve up, and the results were equally as strong. Frank, my head trainer/coach, was convinced my foot problem stemmed from a constrained hip area, so he worked on the area with a vengeance. At the start of each session, my ailing leg was at least an inch shorter than my relatively healthy one. After Frank was done Sticking me, my legs were equal in length. And I'd nearly bitten a hole through a towel to keep from uttering expletives.

The Stick is just one of the wonder tools at a runner's disposal, either for use by yourself or in the hands of a professional. To introduce you to the entire toolbox, brew yourself a cup of herbal tea, slip on a robe, and please join us at the Another Mother Runner Spa.

Picture a young, impossibly beautiful receptionist who talks in a lilting-yet-hushed voice: *Welcome to Another Mother Runner Spa. You've been working really hard, I can tell. Now it's time to step back and to let go. We've got just the restorative treatment for you. Take your time with our menu and figure out what will refresh, rejuvenate, and revitalize you.*

Menu of Services

ACUPUNCTURE

When: Injured

Frequency: Once or twice a week for several weeks, depending on injury

Despite the use of needles, which honestly doesn't hurt, this alternative medicine treatment has a surprisingly calming effect on both healthy and injured runners. At the hands of a talented practitioner, the insertion and manipulation of the needles improves circulation and sends "chi," the healing life force, to the affected area.[1]

$50 to $150

ADVIL, ALEVE, AND OTHER NONSTEROIDAL ANTI-INFLAMMATORY DRUGS

When: Pain sets in

Frequency: Every 3 to 4 hours, or every 12 for Aleve

As the name of this treatment indicates, these are drugs that relieve inflammation and alleviate pain. The label says pop two pills for pain after, say, a long run, but we find it takes three to ease the ouch. They can upset some runners' stomachs, and taken long term, these types of drugs can be hard on the kidneys, so use sparingly. Try wearing your day-after soreness with pride instead.

$4 and up (opt for the jumbo bottle at Costco at the start of marathon training)

---

[1]Sorry to get all woo-woo, but it worked wonders on my plantar fasciitis.

COMPRESSION WEAR

When: After a hard or long workout

Frequency: After every tough session, if so inclined

This category of items consists of snug tights, capris, shorts, calf sleeves, and socks designed to be tight enough to enhance blood flow from your feet and lower legs. The scientific community isn't in agreement about whether these Lycra-laden garments aid performance, so we offer this treatment for recovery only, recommending wearing them after a long run or speedwork, or while you slumber. If you insist on wearing the socks *while* you run, we insist you rock them with a sassy skirt.

$20 to $150

HEAT

When: 15 to 20 minutes as soreness indicates

Frequency: Once or twice a day when suffering

The heat treatment, in the form of a heating pad or hot bath or shower, can be applied before a run to warm up a tight, stiff area. It can also be used a few hours post-sweat to provide pain relief and minimize stiffness on chronically sore back or joint pain, but don't pour on the warmth immediately after exercise.

About $10 for a heating pad

ICE

When: After an acute injury or on a chronic one

Frequency: Three to four times per day for 15 minutes

Part of the therapy known as RICE (Rest, Ice, Compression, Elevation),[1] this element reduces swelling and pain when applied to an acute injury, such as a sprained or strained muscle. No need for a fancy pack: Here at the Another Mother Runner Spa, we utilize bags of frozen vegetables that are, of course, organic. Remove ice or veggies once numbness sets in. This treatment can also be used for a chronic injury, such as plantar fasciitis, to manage inflammation.

Free to $2.69

---

[1]Rest: self-explanatory. Compression: Wrap an ACE bandage around the injured area or wear a compression garment, such as socks, if ankle is sprained. Elevation: Raise the injured area while icing or afterward.

ICE BATH

When: Within an hour after a demanding workout (a double-digit run or other especially strenuous efforts)

Frequency: As often as you can tolerate, after said demanding workout

Begin this treatment by undressing from the waist down, and donning warm, dry clothing up top, such as a fleece jacket and hat. A mug of hot chai or cocoa is recommended, as the mug warms your hands, and the beverage, your belly. Fill the tub with cold water and add the equivalent of one or two 5-pound bags of ice. Then step into the tub and lower your body into the frigid water. If necessary, add more water; the water should come to your hip bones so your legs are completely covered. Sit in the icy concoction, letting it work its restorative magic. After 10 to 20 minutes, get out and take a hot shower. Your beet-red legs will thank you as lactic acid is flushed out of your muscles and inflammation is minimized.

A little H_2O and ice, but mostly free, as suffering doesn't cost a thing

MASSAGE

When: Sore post-workout or injured

Frequency: An hour-long one, as often as budget allows

One of our top-tier treatments, massage seems like a luxury. But for mother runners aiming to set a personal best in a 13.1- or 26.2-mile race, an hour on the table, where your healing blood flows freely and your muscles relax, can make a big difference in a training cycle. Our Mother Runner massage therapists don't travel, so research one in your area: Call a running store or ask a physical therapist for suggestions. A talented therapist will get to know your body, apply the correct amount of pressure, and can sense an impending overuse injury, instead of merely giving you an expensive back rub.

$45 to $90

PAIN-RELIEVING CREAMS

When: Whenever soreness soars

Frequency: As often as you like

When sore, over-run muscles cry out, the answer might be rubbing a pain-relieving cream or gel on them. FlexPower Active Woman is an AMR Spa favorite. This odorless cream, and others like it, creates a warming sensation in muscles, ideal for alleviating pain for several hours or a chemically induced warm-up. For clients (wo)man enough, it can be applied before taking a shower; the hot water increases the cream's intensity by quite a bit. There are also creams and sprays, such as Biofreeze, that provide a cooling sensation. Arnica, a holistic ingredient in gels available at natural-food stores, is an alternative for those who want simple pain relief, not temperature swings. Caution: Do not put counter-irritant creams like these on acute injuries, as they can aggravate inflammation.

About $20

PEDICURE

When: Appropriate when your heels resemble a hunk of Parmesan

Frequency: Whenever you can sneak away

This treatment is ideal for camouflaging discolored toenails[1]: smoothing and buffing calloused, well-worn feet; relaxing; and catching up on six-month-old *People* magazines. Although we recommend silvery OPI Gone Platinum polish to pretty up your tootsies and make you feel as invincible as steel, feel free to pick any color that suits your fancy.

$25 to $40

REST

When: Year-round, but especially during focused training

Frequency: Once or twice per week

This hands-off procedure involves not exercising over the course of 48 hours. Usually done the day before or after a hard effort, rest lets you summon energy stores and permits muscles to recover. Please remember, muscles only get stronger when they are allowed to rebuild during times of rest; too much work and not enough rest lead to lethargy and discontentment, a condition known as cranky mother runner.

Free (although it can be tough to find)

---

[1]Public service announcement: Your running shoes should be at least a half-size larger than your flats, boots, and heels.

DOWNWARD *Dog* LIKE A MOTHER
SIX BEST RECOVERY YOGA POSES

Seeing that pretty much every movement we do in yoga class could be dubbed Awkward, Twisted Pretzel Pose, we turned to Sage Rountree—author of *The Athlete's Guide to Yoga* and *The Athlete's Guide to Recovery*, and a marathon mom of two daughters—for expert advice on the must-do poses for runners. (And if you want more, we love Sage's DVD, *The Athlete's Guide to Yoga*.)

CHILD'S POSE Kneeling, rest your belly on your thighs, your head on (or toward) the floor, and your arms stretched out in front of you. Enjoy noticing your breath on your legs as you release your ankles, quads, hamstrings, and back.

HAPPY BABY Lying on your back, bend your knees and draw them toward your armpits, lifting your feet toward the ceiling in an upside-down squat. Hold the backs of your legs and, if you're feeling very happy, rock right and left. You'll be releasing your back and inner thigh muscles, as well as a smile.

RECLINING FISH AND COBBLER Lie back with a rolled blanket or stack of pillows running the length of your spine. Spread your arms to the side for a chest stretch, so your body forms a T. Put the soles of your feet together and drop your bent knees to either side to stretch your inner thighs.

RECLINING CROSS-LEGGED TWIST Lying on your back, cross your right knee tight over the left and drop both knees to the left, rolling way up onto the outer left hip. Spread your right arm off to the right and breathe, feeling the stretch in your chest, spine, and hips. Repeat on the other side.

LEGS UP THE WALL Sit one hip very close to the wall and take your hands behind you as you swing both legs up, propping your heels over your hips and spreading your arms to the sides. Your butt will be on or near the wall. Relax your back into the floor and enjoy the inversion, which drains swelling in your legs and helps you recover. (This pose is especially great after a race.)

CORPSE POSE Lie flat on your back, palms up, legs slightly separated and toes flopped out, and simply breathe. And pretend you can't hear the cries of, "Mom! Mom! Where are you, Mom?"

REVERSE TAPER

When: The days, weeks, or even month after a race

Frequency: After every race[1]

This critical post-race recovery treatment is too often skipped by enthusiastic runners who immediately resume a regular exercise routine. Instead of picking up where you left off and continuing to tax your body, repeat the week's training leading up to race day—but in reverse. For example, if you ran 6 miles on Sunday, 4 on Tuesday, 3 on Wednesday, and 2 on Thursday before a Saturday race, do 2 on Monday, 3 on Tuesday, 4 on Thursday, and 6 on Saturday. All at a super-relaxed pace. (And if that feels like too much, no pressure: You can cut those miles in half, walk them, or crosstrain.)

For a marathon, many experts recommend taking it easy for a day for every mile of the marathon (we're talking nearly a month). We encourage you to take off the first week post-'thon. Walk if you want and run a little, if you feel like it, but generally give yourself time to recover, clean your closet, get out the dog hair from the corners of the living room, and cook healthy dinners. Then, depending on how you're feeling, you can start to run again, slowly and short distances only. Two weeks post-marathon, you can reverse your taper, as explained above.

Free (and you'll thank us for it afterward)

ROLFING

When: Your whole body feels like it needs to push the reset button

Frequency: Ten consecutive sessions, done weekly or every other week

This comprehensive body treatment involves both a significant time and financial commitment. A series of 10 structured sessions realigns the fascia, or connective tissue of the body, so that your body can function the way Mother Nature intended—not as your stride, posture, and lifestyle have morphed it to be. Each session focuses on "organizing" a specific body element: the area around your rib cage, the length of your backside, the leg from the ankle to the pelvis. The pressure can be significantly more intense than a massage, but for Dimity, the results were definitely worth the pain and expense.

Approximately $100/session; find a certified Rolfer at Rolf.org

---

[1] Caveat: This treatment should not be followed after a see-how-things-feel race done as part of a buildup to a target race—for example, a 10K that's part of training for a marathon. In that case, ease back into a training plan 2 or 3 days post-race.

TAKE IT *From* A MOTHER
ARE YOU A SERIAL RACER/TRAINER, A MOSTLY RUN-FOR-FUN'ER, OR SOMEWHERE IN BETWEEN?

"A bit of both. I really love to be on a training schedule, but I also really enjoy the few weeks after a race when I run for pleasure."

—ALLYSON (Runs at 6 A.M.-ish because she "loves to be done.")

"I like to schedule workouts, and I do better while on a training plan. I am currently winging it and am struggling with the lack of structure."

—EMILY (Dreams of a running date with Vin Diesel. "But only if he doesn't talk.")

"Having a future race goal gives my workouts meaning and keeps me motivated, so I schedule at least one race a month."

—LAURA (Improves her speed with "Dirty 30s": "Go at an easy pace for 30 steps, then at sprint pace for 30 steps. Repeat several times.")

"As far as training, I do my own thing. I called my last marathon training the 'Leslie Slacker Training Plan,' and I ran a PR. But I am a serial racer. It's only May, and I'm already working on my racing schedule for next year."

—LESLIE (Tracks her race times on Athlinks.com.)

"Over the years, I have gone back and forth. Right now, I'm in serious training mode, but I think 'down' times, when you run for the joy of running, are important."

—TERZAH (Forgot her bra for the NYC Marathon but didn't realize her error until the morning of the race. Thankfully, she borrowed one from a friend. "I'm pretty flat chested, but not flat enough that I wanted to run braless for 26. 2 miles.")

"After every race, I tell myself 'After this race, I'm taking time off.' Then, the little voice in my head tells me to sign up for something else."

—MELISSA (Didn't realize the Ziploc bag holding her Clif Shot Bloks—and stored in her shorts liner—had a hole in it until mile 12 of a marathon. "I grabbed a cup of Gatorade, dumped it out, dug out the Bloks, put them in the cup, and used the Bloks. Not a proud moment in my life.")

"It's always about the next race."

—HEATHER (Races in her dad's "ratty and faded" Phillies visor. "He died suddenly, and I need him with me during races.")

SELF-MASSAGE

When: Preferably after most runs or when aches make themselves known

Frequency: Daily, whenever possible

One of our most reasonably priced offerings, self-massage is performed by your hands or tools you already possess. Feeling tight in your quadriceps or a twinge in your Achilles tendon? Reach in and search out the sore spot. Trace it back to its origin, seeing if mild to moderate pressure there helps alleviate tension. Self-massage helps release knots and adhesions in soft tissue like muscles and fascia.

As noted previously, this treatment can also be done with a variety of tools. Many of our clients swear by rolling out tight IT bands, cramped gluteal muscles, and even impinged shoulders on a foam roller, for instance, after every run or every evening. Others keep a golf ball under their desk to roll their arch throughout the workday. You can even take a rolling pin to your legs, substituting your legs for dough as you roll. Even a few minutes are beneficial in (and *on*) the long run.

Free

SLEEP

When: Not too long after your kids hit the hay

Frequency: Every night, and sometimes in the afternoon

The most restorative of all recovery aids, sleep is also the one most often ignored. It may sound like a shocking amount, but the body needs 7 to 9 hours every night to bring back vitality. Sleep experts recommend supplementing this standard based on how many miles per week you are running. Add as many minutes per night as miles you run in a week. Stacking up 25 miles this week in anticipation of your fall half-marathon? Spend 25 more minutes in slumber per night or in the form of a nap. As accommodating as we like to be at AMR Spa, we don't have a way to provide this extra time to you. But we recommend not answering all your e-mail, not being fastidious about every crumb on the kitchen counter, and not picking up after children who are old enough to do it themselves.

Free (although sometimes it feels you pay dearly for ordering this treatment)

STRETCHING

When: After a workout

Frequency: As often as is convenient

Still a highly debated subject—Should I stretch before or after I run? Should I go lightly or deeply?—stretching is a treatment that should be guided by your body. Releasing the tension from your muscles after a run can be nirvana, but go gently: A hamstring stretch shouldn't bring tears to your eyes. Be sure to hit your hips and glutes (the classic figure-4 stretch—crossing an ankle over one thigh, then sitting back as in a chair—is a good one) as well as your quads, hamstrings, and calves.

Free (and you accrue AMR Spa reward points if your children or dogs crawl on top of you while you stretch)

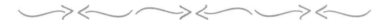

.1   ARE YOU WITH ME?
By Sarah

A few hours after my first husband made the abrupt, out-of-the-blue announcement that he wanted out of our marriage, I asked him if he would still accompany me to the out-of-state triathlon I was doing the following month. *Please.* Yes, amid my torrent of tears and body-racking sobs, I knew I wouldn't be able to ply the lake or run along the country roads unless John was there to support me, even if our marriage was the emotional equivalent of a flat tire. It's hard for me to imagine now, but at the time, I had to have him at every athletic event I did—be it rowing in the Head of the Charles Regatta or running a 10K along San Francisco's Embarcadero—otherwise I'd feel too nervous and weak. (Me? I know, hard to imagine. But true.)

Fast forward a mere four years, after I'd limped through the unexpected divorce and the resulting emotional fallout to land squarely on my own two feet. Jack had achieved live-in boyfriend status, and I was immersed in training for the New York City Marathon. We lived in San Francisco, and I'd bought my plane tickets to the Big Apple months earlier. I was out for drinks with gal pals a month or so pre-NYC when one of them asked if Jack was going with me. I snorted Hefeweizen out my nose. Jack go to watch me run the marathon? It was a laughable suggestion: Why on earth did I need my man there? I was capable and excited all on my own, thank you very much.

The topic didn't even come up between Jack and me until about ten days before I was due to jet east. By that point, a ticket would have cost a king's ransom and, again, what was the point? It honestly didn't occur to me until *after* the marathon that it might have been special for Jack to see me push myself in a running race, but I didn't feel any burning need to have him there for support. I'd toughened up and learned how to fly—and run—solo. Funny how a thing like divorce will do that to a gal.

I'd also become a more competent, confident athlete. Navigating a race expo or jockeying for a spot in a starting corral didn't intimidate me like it had in the married-to-John days when I was a race novice. Now I gained courage and pride by going it alone. It added to my sense of accomplishment: I came, I saw, I conquered. Just me. Nobody else.

Even now I rarely ask Jack, and the other, shorter spectators in our house, to come to my races. I understand it's a huge hassle to load them all up, find parking, get them to the right spot, then entertain them for what feels like—and can be—hours until I show up for a millisecond. But for the 2010 Portland Marathon, with my heart set on running fast enough to qualify for the Boston Marathon, I asked my cheering section to be there. My weekend training runs often took me down a long stretch of the course, and I'd envisioned my family foursome under a large sugar maple near the 21-mile mark, or, in other words, prime wall-hitting territory. I was so intent on them being under that *specific* tree, I drove Jack by it twice and wrote down the address of the house it was in front of. And to ensure there was no mistake, no, "Oh, she doesn't really care if we watch her run or not," ambiguity, a few nights before the race, I told Jack in my most solemn, I-mean-it voice, "If you don't show up at the marathon, I. Will. Never. Forget. It."

I don't know why it felt so important for them to be there. Maybe a part of me is envious when I see all the adorable, kid-made "Go, Mom," "Mommy Runners Rock!" and, of course, "Run Like a Mother" signs other mother runners post on our Facebook page. I knew my brood wouldn't have any signs, but I figured my twins + cowbells = a loud racket.

Come race day, rain was falling in sheets, as a part of me had predicted it would, thus the pre-race suggestion of the leafy canopy to serve as nature's umbrella. Rounding a bend in the course, I spied my huddled masses under the appointed tree. A smile burst onto my face, and my steps felt lighter. Sure, my son, John, barely registered me when I briefly stopped to hand them an empty water bottle and to babble something idiotic like, "Weather sucks, huh?" but I got a major boost from seeing them.

As I continued toward the finish line, I thought about how I am strong enough to go it alone now, but that sometimes it's nice to know I don't have to. Funny how life works out like that.

10

INJURIES: THE FIVE STAGES OF GRIEF

By Dimity

The pain started about mid-June. Little pinpricks would light up across the top of my right foot after a run. It was a novel pain, delicate and interesting, but not debilitating. I kept going; I had my eyes on the 2010 New York City Marathon. Within a few weeks, the pinpricks turned to lightning bolts, which struck most intensely when I wore my silver flip-flops post-run. Some people would stop wearing the shoes, but I loved those silver flip-flops, which matched every-thing and were trendy—another novelty for my hard-to-fit feet. So I wore them and pretended I wasn't being shocked with each step. By early August, my foot felt like a Fourth of July night sky. Still, I kept running, albeit for shorter distances. I also switched shoes, tried to change my form, walked barefoot when I walked our dogs to encourage my feet to return to their natural state, and wished the pain would simply decide one day to disappear. Because, you know, run-ning injuries typically do that.

Having lived in my body for almost 40 years, though, I knew better. While procrastinating during the day, I'd Google "top of foot pain" and "running"—I didn't want to put the words *stress fracture* into the universe, even though I was 90 percent sure that was what I was dealing with—and click on links until I'd see those dreaded two words and immediately close the window. Not only was I in an empire state of mind, I also had a couple of running commitments (pacing my ultrarunning friend Katie for about 11 miles in the Leadville Trail 100, pacing my pal Pip in a 5K) that I simply couldn't stomach missing. Unlike my first stress fracture three years prior, which was in my left heel and which I couldn't ignore unless I was lying flat on my back, this one was less intense. The fireworks eventually settled into a constant bee sting that, while far from comfortable, wasn't unbearable.

TAKE IT *From* A MOTHER
HAVE YOU (TRIED TO) RUN THROUGH INJURY?

"In a 5K, every step was painful. I felt like I was running grueling 15-minute miles; shin splints had taken over. I recovered with ice packs and chiropractic care."
—MEGAN (Worst night before a race: sharing a bed with her sideways-sleeping, kicking son.)

"My SI joint flared up a mile away from home, and I couldn't bear weight through my leg. I am a physical therapist, so I lay down in the road and attempted to correct it, but I couldn't fix it without assistance. I had to hobble home, and it took 2 weeks to recover. My husband jokes the only reason I became a PT was to treat my own injuries."
—CHRISTY (Proudest running moment: making state all 4 years in high school track.)

"I had hairline fractures in both shins, but it took awhile to get a diagnosis. I ran a 21-mile run on the fractures but was unable to complete marathon training. Now I get new shoes every 400 miles, and I don't push myself beyond my limits."
—COURTNEY (Next on her running list of things to do: speedwork.)

"Yes. In the weeks leading up to my first half-marathon, I was having extreme leg and hip pain. The elliptical didn't seem to aggravate it, so I did that. I survived the race, but could barely walk 15 minutes later."
—MELISSA (Compulsive about ending her runs on a whole number. "I'll run a lap around a parking lot to make sure I don't end at 6.95 miles.")

"No. I've had two stress fractures, and during the first one, I realized I could crosstrain. So when it happened again, I knew there were other things I could do, and it would feel so much better to get out there when it's fully healed."
—TRACY (Started running after her third daughter was stillborn. "I needed a way to channel my emotions.")

"I developed tendonitis in my ankle from running on uneven snow. My PT had me run without shoes and set a metronome to speed up my turnover, and my stride evened out. He treated the tendonitis, and I started running in Saucony Kinvaras at 180 steps per minute. Totally changed my running."
—KIM (Found her BRF when a woman stopped her car and got out and asked to talk to her during a run. "I thought she wanted directions, but she wanted a running partner.")

But it wasn't going away, and after I ran next to my friends—I didn't tell either until we were in the thick of the races, because I didn't want them to worry about me—I knew I had to really stop. An X-ray and examination confirmed what I already knew: I was officially injured. When the orthopedist said I'd have to wear a boot and sent his nurse to get one, I said I already had one. Although I had wanted to toss that black monstrosity after stress fracture numero uno, I had buried it in a far-flung closet in case I needed it for a Halloween costume. That night, I asked Grant to get it for me, and as soon as I saw it, I got the feeling of having a piece of dry toast stuck in my throat. I could hardly breathe.

I was already weary of the late-August, mid-90s temperatures, and knowing I had to clomp around in a hot, hefty boot for 6 weeks was simply too much. My breathing returned, but the tears started pouring. I Velcro'd on the inner boot, which was festooned with dog hair and tiny balls of lint, and through sobs, I fastened on the clompy part that would keep my foot still enough to heal. I kept the Frankenfoot on for the better part of 7 weeks. I pushed the gas pedal with it; I went camping wearing it; I wore it out to dinner on date night. (The doc told me to sleep in it. No. Just no.)

As I went through the 5-month ordeal, I realized I was living the five steps of grief, a process of dealing with death that was introduced by psychiatrist Elisabeth Kübler-Ross in her 1969 book, *On Death and Dying*. I wasn't grieving in the most despondent sense—my family was healthy, my husband and I were employed, there was no imminent tragedy—but a running injury is much more traumatic than the physical ailment. For most of us, running is so much more than the act of putting one foot in front of the other. It's an elixir for self-definition, empowerment, endorphins, strength, deep thoughts, joy, and confidence. Take away my run, and my life does a seismic shift in the wrong direction.

Bearing that in mind—and to validate your feelings next time you're knocked out—I present to you the five stages of running-injury grief.

STAGE 1: DENIAL AND ISOLATION

You're in this stage if: Your thought about your IT band syndrome, shin splints, or other malady is that it truly isn't a problem. "It doesn't really hurt when I stand this way," you tell yourself, shifting all your weight to the noninjured side. "When I run only on trails and not more than 2 miles every third day, I'm totally fine," you say to a friend. "Totally fine."

In other words, you don't accept you're hurt—or are on your way to being the sidelined kind of injured—so you keep running and tweaking your form in search of the pain-free run. In defense of our often delusional brains, it could be very likely that the new state of pain or your compromised gait is the only reality you know. As I've described too many times, I had piercing pain in my left hip and glute for almost 3 years, and it just became a way of life: I put on my jeans sitting on the bed so I didn't have to balance on my gimpy left leg.

Once the pain makes itself undeniably known or a doctor gives you a get-real diagnosis, you realize something has to give. But you can't conceive of a life without running: How are you ever going to get to (or afford) the gym? And if you do get there, what are you going to do? Get on the elliptical and stare at somebody's back for an hour? Ugh.

True Stage 1 example: Flying with SBS last spring, I noticed she hobbled like a rodeo cowboy as we deplaned together. I didn't think this 1-MPH walk was fodder for a joke, so I asked if she was okay. "Yeah, it's just my ankle and heel," said Sarah, always an optimist. "Doesn't that happen to you when you've been sitting for a long time?" I chose not to answer because, no, I don't usually look like I need a skycap with a wheelchair when I get off an airplane.

Two days later, she ran a half-marathon, then finally allowed herself to accept that her case of plantar fasciitis was nastier than she wanted it to be, and that the only way to kill that sucker was to take a break from her beloved sport. (BTW, if jealousy were part of the stages, it would enter in here for me: In 28 years of running, that was the *first* injury-related break she's ever had to take. Yeah, I know. You can be jealous, too.)

STAGE 2: ANGER

You're in this stage if: Your mood can best be described as bitchy, crabby, or irate. You might be pissed at your running friends. You guys were all training for the same half-marathon, using the exact, down-to-the-very-last-step plan. How can all three of them still be running happy while you're sitting in a doctor's waiting room? Or, at the gas station, you might shoot a scowl at some random stranger who is wearing a pair of running shoes and a Lycra-infused outfit that indicates he might have logged some miles in the last few hours.

Chances are, though, your loved ones are the ones in your bull's-eye; just as kids can be perfect for a babysitter and have a total meltdown when you step one foot inside the door, you can put on a brave face for the world and peel off the plastic when you're at home. You may be snippy to your husband, who simply does not get why taking something, especially something physically taxing, *off* your to-do list is grounds for such self-pity. And when he splurges to surprise you and cheer you up with dinner from the Whole Foods prepared-food section, you're incredulous. "Really? Häagen-Dazs peanut butter and chocolate ice cream for dessert? Why don't you just paste it right on my thighs?"

While you're likely more compassionate toward your children, your normal level of patience has left the building. "Didn't I tell you to pick up your backpack?" you bellow twice in a 30-second span at your child, who just walked in the door from school and beelined to the bathroom.

You might even get angry with your own body. You may step on the scale more times than is healthy, or decide that today is the day you're going to nail the one-hundred-push-up program, but because you can't run, and crave sweat and burn, you opt to start on Day 14, not Day 1.

True Stage 2 example: Like your body getting used to the feeling your IT band is as tightly strung as the shortest string on a harp, your mood can get so used to this emotional state that it simply always surrounds you, like the dirt perpetually engulfing Pig-Pen. I could write entire novels about how I take out my frustration on my family (and likely make you feel better about your actions), but suffice it to say, I am not always the nice person I appear to be in public.

After an MRI revealed two bulging discs and a severely arthritic back—yet another hash mark in my injury column—the doctor suggested I try Pilates. I did, and about a year later, at approximately the same time of night I would've likely been pissed at Grant because he had, once again, forgotten to put out the recycling and garbage, I asked him if he thought I was standing taller. His response to that question was lukewarm, but then he added, "But you haven't complained about your body and how much it hurts in months. That's worth so much, I'd subsidize Pilates for the rest of your life." (Please note: He speaks well, but he has not yet subsidized any of my Pilates. I pay for that out of my own account, not our joint funds.)

PRACTICAL *Motherly* ADVICE
TYPICAL INJURY CAUSES AND CURES

Unlike running injuries, where we tend to ignore our limits ("Oh, this piercing pain in my glute isn't anything"), we know our boundaries when it comes to doling out advice about injuries. We are far from being physical therapists or doctors, yet we know that injuries are squirrely little suckers. Out-of-whack hips, an overambitious stride, or roughly 736 other factors can cause an angry knee.

So we asked Janet Hamilton, an excellent exercise physiologist and running coach, the author of *Running Strong & Injury Free*, and the mother to two golden retrievers, to help define the most common causes and cures for widespread injuries. Please note: The cures work only if you actually ice, stretch, do your strength work, scale back your miles, and so forth—and not just read about doing so.

SHIN SPLITS

What it feels like: Tenderness on or alongside the shin bone

How you got them: Ramping up your mileage too fast, going a little overboard at the track, or some combo thereof; excessive pronation, or your feet rolling inward when you land; inadequate hip strength and core strength; worn-out shoes, or a sudden change to shoes with less support than you're used to.

What can help: Ice; gentle and frequent stretching of the calf muscles; orthotics if needed (either over-the-counter or prescription); scaling back your miles and avoiding hills until you feel better; hip-strengthening exercises, especially lunges in all directions (forward, backward, side to side).

ACHILLES TENDONITIS

What it feels like: The area above your heel and behind your anklebones is tender and sore. The soreness can sneak up on you, and if you catch it before it becomes more pronounced, you can save yourself months of rehab.

How you got it: Wearing shoes that don't give you the amount of support you need (could be that there's either too little, or too much, guidance); supertight calves; weak hips (we don't blame you; we blame the kids you carried); not being smart about increasing your training intensity (you deserve a little blame here).

What can help: Icing after running, orthotics, eccentric exercises like heel drops,[1] dramatically scaling back your runs, or taking breaks. Heel lifts, used in both shoes, might provide temporary relief, but don't rely on them long term.

PLANTAR FASCIITIS

What it feels like: A pain in the bottom of the heel or in the arch, which is most apparent either first thing in the morning or when you stand up from being seated. It usually gets better as you move around.

How you got it: Calf muscles are wound tighter than your boss; your shoes don't have enough support; going too far or too fast without giving your body time to catch up; making a sudden change in terrain, speed, footwear, or running form.

---

[1]Stand on a step on the balls of both feet, weight balanced, then press up so your heels are above the step. Then shift all your weight to your injured leg, and slowly lower the heel so it is even with the step. Do 10 to 25, and incrementally allow your heel to drop below the step.

What can help: Rolling a golf or tennis ball, or a frozen water bottle, under your foot for 10 to 15 minutes once or twice a day; wearing a resting night splint or specially designed strap that keeps your foot flexed overnight; gently but frequently stretching your calves; getting in the right shoes with the right amount of support for you; backing off the mileage and intensity work, as well as hills; and working on hip strength. (Yep, note the theme: The butt is connected to the foot.)

ILIOTIBIAL BAND FRICTION SYNDROME (ITBS)

What it feels like: A pain in the outside of your knee and possibly in the lower thigh.

How you got it: Excessive pronation; weak hips and glutes; tight calves, hamstrings, or quads.

What can help: Strengthening your hips (Google "clamshell exercise for hips" to find a demonstration); stretching tight calves or hamstrings; self-massage with a foam roller or other device; new shoes; massage.

RUNNER'S KNEE

What it feels like: A whiny knee, which is felt most acutely after a run; when you sit for long periods of time (driving 2 hours to Grandma's house or sitting through a movie); or when you go up and down stairs.

How you got it: Inadequate hip strength (yes, that culprit again!); feet that pronate too far and aren't being supported with the right type of footwear; tight hamstrings and calves.

What can help: Strengthening your hips and quads; stretching; ice; orthotics or a change in footwear; a great sports massage (yeah, we know: as if you have the time—or funds—for it).

STRESS FRACTURE

What it feels like: Localized bruiselike pain on a bone that causes you to wince when you push on it; it may hurt even at rest.

How you got it: Biomechanical issues; low bone-mineral density; underfueling; ramping up mileage or intensity too quickly; sudden changes in terrain, footwear, or gait pattern; inadequate rest.

What can help: Time off to let the bone heal (expect between 6 to 8 weeks); crosstraining if you have no pain in the injured area; focused strength training that can help support the area when you do get back to running.

STAGE 3: BARGAINING

You're in this stage if: All your thoughts with regard to running and your injury involve an if/then statement.

- If I can run this 10K in 2 weeks, then I'll stop running after the race and really allow myself to get better.

- If I can hire a coach to help me change my form, then I'll never get hurt again.

- If I can get a cortisone shot (or two), then I'll be able to get through the marathon.

- If only I can hunt down those special shoes that everybody on the Internet is raving about, then I'll be on my way to recovery.

- If I diligently use my foam roller every morning and night—and maybe even sleep with it next to me so I can jump on it when a kid wakes me up at 2:00 A.M.—then my hip flexor will relax once and for all.

- If I ditch my shoes and run barefoot all the time, then my Morton's neuroma will disappear.

- If I honor my body by eating more soy, kale, and chia seeds and less caffeine, sugar, and gluten, then my body will honor me and, in return, heal my Achilles tendon.

True Stage 3 example: Sarah's plantar fasciitis had an acute onset: During her final pre-race track workout, within the first few steps of her sixth 800-meter repeat, it was as if she had stepped on a metal spike that drove up into her right heel. A half-marathon was a mere five days away. Never having been injured before—like I said, total envy is expected and normal—she was unsure how it would all play out. Her more immediate concern was how she'd get home: Putting any pressure on her right foot was excruciating. Visions of crawling the half-mile home filled her head; she debated whether she could hobble home like a three-legged dog. After much teeth gnashing and many deep breaths, she was able to stand upright and limp along the sidewalk. Her usual 5-minute jaunt took nearly 20 minutes.

Delusional and in deep denial, she thought maybe it would be serviceable by race day. Her first vow was to not run on it again until the race. (*If I don't run on it until race day, then it'll be just fine!*) In the next few days, as she began to grasp the scope of the problem, her mind scrambled with bargains. The one she kept coming back to: "If I can make it through the race without hearing—or feeling—a big 'pop' or 'snap,' then I'll take time off." After asking a race official the protocol for dropping out midrace in the point-to-point course, Sarah unwisely covered the 13.1 miles. Adrenaline must have masked the pain, which she ranked at a 2 or 3 during the race; moments after the finish line, it shot up to a 9. It took the two us nearly as long to return to our hotel (.4 miles from the start) as it did for her to run the course, and the grimace on her face far outshone her finisher's medal.

STAGE 4: DEPRESSION

You're in this stage if: You have completely and totally given in to your injury—and given up on being active. It's hard to remember why running brought you any pleasure. When you see a runner on the road, you're no longer angry with them. Instead, you just think they're wasting their time. "Why bother if you're only going to get injured?" you think.

If you've been prescribed certain physical therapy exercises to help you heal, you do them half as often as you're supposed to. Or maybe you don't even do that. Your foam roller is collecting dust. You may bail on some massage or acupuncture appointments, since your improvement seems so minor compared with the cash you're laying out. Any thoughts of sneaking into your race, if you had one on the horizon, are definitely squelched. You sleep in more than you know you should, shower less than you know you should, and watch more shows on Bravo while consuming more Dove Bars than you know you should.

True Stage 4 example: I should be sponsored by Kleenex based on the number of boxes I've gone through while crying about running injuries. Most of those tears were shed solo. As in I wasn't even talking to anybody. I was simply sad and alone, and I couldn't get my run on to not feel so sad and alone.

A certain patina settled over me when I hit this stage of my second round of boot wearing. Things were different. The first time, I was able to keep training on the bike (see page 156) and run the 2007 Nike Women's Marathon 6 weeks after removing the boot. The second time, I didn't have the mojo to spend the equivalent of at least a cumulative week on the bike to run another marathon. So I had no prize to eye. Because I wasn't really sweating, and because the boot was a pain to disassemble, I minimized my showers. The circles under my eyes must have been unusually murky, because when I met SBS in San Francisco to speak, ironically, at the 2010 Nike Women's Marathon, our first stop was at Benefit to get me some makeup, including under-eye concealer. What's more, I felt fat—and should've, given how I was eating. A huge bowl of leftover Annie's Mac & Cheese, two pieces of toast covered in butter, and three chocolate chip cookies is a good lunch for a sedentary person, right?

TAKE IT *From* A MOTHER
WHAT'S THE BEST SIGN YOU'VE SEEN ON RACE DAY?[1]

"You made it to the start. You will make it to the finish."

—AMANDA (Her family members position themselves a bit before the finish, so they will see her coming in strong without a lot of people in the way.)

"Keep running. People are watching."

—LISA (During family fun runs, sticks with her husband until the last half-mile, when she completely blows him away.)

"Do or do not. There is no try. —Yoda"

—KATIE (Removes her shoes to run in socks if her feet start hurting.)

"Lisa #26372: Donnie Wahlberg is waiting at the finish line naked with crab sauce and cannoli cake."

—LISA (Named her basement treadmill Donnie Wahlberg because "It's fun to get on him and get a workout.")

"In front of a church: 'Is there a patron saint of blisters?' and 'Even atheists pray at mile 24.'"

—PATTY (Has run two "huge" PRs in the two races she wore her "Badass Mother Runner" shirt—which are available at anothermotherrunner.com . . . just sayin'.)

"Hello complete stranger. I'm so proud of you."

—STEPHANIE (Looks forward to Tuesday-night dates with the TV [to watch *Glee*] and treadmill [to do speedwork].)

"Pain is temporary. Your time will be posted on the Internet forever!"

—DANIELLE (On training runs, has an iPod on her arm, headlamp on her head, reflective vest with a rear light attached, and pepper spray in her hand. Plus, house key and phone. "I'm trying to figure out what I'm going to do when I start doing longer runs and need water and GUs. I should bring the wagon.")

---

[1]We deliberately put this in the injury chapter for two reasons: First, for comic relief. Second, for inspiration, in case you're up for being a spectator and helping others get through their races.

> *"That hill is your bitch."*
>
> —AMANDA (Introvert or extrovert on race day? "I smack strangers on the ass. If it looks really good, I'll grab.")
>
> *"My sister held a sign once in the Chicago half-marathon: 'Hurry up! I'm FREEZING!'"*
>
> —SUSAN (Loves hearing "Go Mom!" during a race. "I'll feed off that even if it's not my family.")
>
> *"DID YOU POOP?"*
>
> —DARCY (Coincidentally, happens to have poop anxiety. "I MUST poop before a race.")
>
> *"No, you're not close, but you're doing great!"*
>
> —TINA (Loves the trails around her Chico, California, home, but avoids them in the summer because of buzz worms, aka rattlesnakes.)
>
> *" F—— this, let's go bowling!"*
>
> —AMY (While on a run saw a lady walking a guinea pig. "It had a little harness and everything.")
>
> *"Go, Mom! (What's for dinner?)"*
>
> —PHOEBE (Saw the sign during a half-marathon on Mother's Day eve.)

STAGE 5: **ACCEPTANCE**

You're in this stage if: You start setting your alarm for 5:30 and get up 4 days a week, just so you're ready to rock when your body is ready to roll. Or when your kids settle into *Good Luck Charlie*, you settle into 20 minutes of clamshell and other less-than-scintillating but very necessary physical-therapy exercises. You start to look up shorter races 5 months away on Active.com, and picture yourself running one of them with no issues. As you begin to eat small crumbs of improvement, you start to encourage others who might be in one of the stages in your rearview mirror.

True Stage 5 example: After seeing a sports-medicine doctor and a podiatrist, and forgoing running completely for a month and a half, SBS fully embraced the full panoply of treatments for her foot. Any cure she read on the Internet, she did. She had acupuncture treatments, religiously took Aleve every morning and evening, rolled her foot on a frozen water bottle several times a day, wore only orthopedically correct footwear, slept in a Strassburg Sock, wore a copper-infused compression brace, and stretched her foot for several minutes before stepping out of bed every morning. She did the "trace the alphabet with your foot" drill so many times, I'm betting her foot writing is easier to read than her 6-year-olds' handwriting.

Despite her diligence, recovery took far longer than she ever would have anticipated when she was struck lame that mid-May morning. Her twins finished their final month of kindergarten, enjoyed their summer vacation, and were filling their backpacks with back-to-school supplies by the time Sarah felt she could say with any certainty that her plantar fasciitis had been tamed into true submission. But she'd learned to accept she had joined the ranks of injured runners—and had, at least once, experienced the five stages of grief that accompany injury.

Pedal LIKE THIS MOTHER
THE MARATHON-READY CYCLING PLAN

By Dimity

When I suffered a stress fracture in my heel about a third of the way through training for the 2007 Nike Women's Marathon, I wasn't ready to quit. I attached my road bike to a trainer and took a trial spin in the basement. My heel didn't hurt. Phew. So I kept training with guidance from a super-resourceful coach, Ivana Bisaro of Carmichael Training Systems.

Since I crossed that finish line, I've probably fielded at least a hundred questions about how I trained for a marathon on a bike—my longest run was 16 miles, pre-marathon—and the answer I always give is, "I worked really hard." I don't consciously hold back specifics; it's just that the details are too complicated to fit in a neat, verbal package. And, to be honest, I don't remember them all that well.

But they fit in this book just fine, so I asked Ivana, who is now a mom to three kids, to grace us with her bike-to-run training knowledge for a runner who is injured during half-marathon training and doesn't want to hang it up. (If you're gunning for a marathon, extend the longer rides on the weekends to the amount of time you'd be running long.)

A few caveats from somebody who has done this before: This is not an easy plan. Be prepared, as I did, to work. Hard. Chances are, it will actually improve your cardiovascular fitness, as it did mine. And it looks complicated, but once you get the hang of things, it's not so confusing. Best of all, this sucker is ridiculously effective. I maintained my sweat-laced sanity, healed my heel, and headed off to San Francisco with fresh legs and a newly rekindled love of running. Oh, and I ran a PR on a crazy hilly course.

BEFORE YOU START

What you need: A heart rate monitor; a road bike with a trainer that attaches to its back wheel (trainer is available at REI or bike stores) or access to a spinning bike (not a recumbent or traditional exercise bike, but one that puts you in a true cycling position); pedals on either style of bike with either cages or clip-in capability—the latter is preferred.

Optional equipment: A $50 iTunes gift card, a new book to listen to, or a TiVo with full seasons of your five favorite shows—in other words, you're going to need some new entertainment; a pool for deep-water running.

With regard to that injury: If your leg, foot, hip, or other injured part hurts when you cycle, you're out. You can't get better if it hurts. Even if it doesn't hurt, do these workouts inside, so you can bail if need be. (Clarification: If your injury, not your heart and lungs, hurt.)

Last bits of advice: Running muscles are not the same as cycling muscles, which your quads may remind you when you hit the bike on the second day. If you haven't been on a bike since middle school, start conservatively; at most, match your long ride to your long run. Finally, a cadence—or the number of revolutions one pedal has in 1 minute—around 90 has the best carryover to running, but it may be hard to get there if you haven't been in the saddle in a while. Don't worry: You'll be there before you know it.

WORKOUT TYPE	HEART RATE[1]	CADENCE[2]	RPE[3]	DESCRIPTION
Endurance (E)	50–91 percent	80+	5	Comfortable endurance pace
Tempo (T)	88–90 percent	70–75	6	A slower cadence that builds leg strength
Steady state (SS)	92–94 percent	80–95	7	Hard effort that increases your aerobic threshold, which is when you go from breathing comfortably to gasping a bit. Scientifically speaking, it's when your body produces more lactic acid—the stuff that causes your muscles to scream when you pick up the pace—than it can clear. Not surprisingly, the amount of time you sustain this pace is limited.
Climbing repeat (CR)	95–97 percent	80–95	8	Threshold work climbing.
Power intervals (PI)	101 percent	90+	10	Maximal effort intervals. Take 30–45 seconds to build up to maximal sustainable power.
One-leg pedal (OLP)	N/A	N/A	5	Drill: With one foot on the pedal, and the other resting on the frame of the bike out of the way, focus on a smooth circular pedal stroke so pulling through bottom and pushing over top.
Fast pedal (FP)	N/A	N/A	5	Drill: Ramp up cadence to maximal sustainable cadence without bouncing in saddle. Keep pedal stroke smooth by pulling through the bottom of the pedal stroke and pushing over the top. Keep upper body relaxed.

1 These numbers come from your higher average heart rate in the field test, which is on Tuesday of Week 1. To find your ranges, multiply that number by the percentages given. For example, if your average heart rates for the tests were 167 and 170 beats per minute, you'd use 170 to calculate your ranges.
Endurance: 50 to 91 percent
Doing the math: 170 x .50 = 85 bpm
              170 x .91 = 154 bpm

2 The number of times your pedals go around in 1 minute. If you don't have a way to electronically track it, count the number of times one foot goes around in 20 seconds, and multiply it by 3. Check in regularly to make sure you're on target.

3 A range from 1 to 10, where 1 is an effort equal to sitting and watching your toddler teeter around on his Skuut bike, and 10 is all out chasing after him because he's about to head down a black diamond–steep hill.

The **BIKE-TO-RUN** Plan

Quick Key:
RBI = Rest between intervals   RBS = Rest between sets

WEEK	MONDAY	TUESDAY	WEDNESDAY	THURSDAY	FRIDAY	SATURDAY	SUNDAY
1	Rest[1]	Field test. E: 50 min., with 15 min. WU; 2 x 8 min. max. efforts with 10 min. RBI[2]	E: 30 min., with OLP 2 sets of 3 x 30 sec.; 7 min. RBS[3]	E: 45 min., with 2 x 8 min. SS; 6 min. RBI.[4]	Rest	E: 75–90 min., with 15 min. T[5]	E: 45 min., with 5 x 60 sec. FP; 60 sec. RBI[6]
2	Rest	E: 60 min., with 3 x 8 min. SS; 6 min. RBI	E: 45 min., with 4 x 60 sec. FP; 60 sec. RBI	E: 60 min., with 2 x 10 min. SS; 6 min. RBI	Rest	90 min., with 2 x 15 min. T; 5 min. RBI	Pool run E: 30 min.[7]
3	Rest	E: 60 min., with 3 x 10 min. SS; 5 min. RBI	Pool run E: 30–45 min	E: 60 min., with 3 x 8 min. SS; 5 min. RBI + 4 x 60 sec. FP; 60 sec. RBI	Rest	E: 100 min., with 25 min. T	E: 45 min., with 2 sets of 3 x 30 sec. OLP; 5 min. RBS
4	Rest	E: 45 min., with 4 x 90 sec. FP; 90 sec. RBI	Rest	E: 45 min., with 30 min. T	Rest	E : 75 min., with two sets of 3 x 45 sec. OLP; 5 min. RBI	Pool run E: 30 min.
5	Rest	E: 60 min., with two sets of 2 x 3 min PI; 3 min. RBI; 10 min. RBS[8]	E: 45 min., with 4 x 90 sec. FP; 60 sec. RBI	E: 60 min. 2 x 8 min. SS; 5 min. RBI; plus 2 x 8 min. CR; 5 min. RBI	Rest	E: 105 min., with two sets of 4 x 45 sec. OLP; 5 min. RBS	Pool run E: 45 min.
6	Rest	E: 60 min., with two sets of 3 x 3 min. PI; 3 min. RBI; 7–10 min. RBS	Pool run E: 45 min.	E: 60 min. with 3 x 8 min. CR; 6 min. RBI	Rest	E: 120 min. EM	E: 45 min., with two sets of 4 x 45 sec. OLP; 5 min. RBS; plus 5 x 60 sec. FP; 60 sec. RBI
7	Rest	E: 60 min., with two sets of 3 x 3 min. PI; 3 min. RBI; 7–10 min. RBS	E: 45 min., with two sets of 3 x 60 sec. OLP; 5 min. RBS	E: 60 min., with 6 x 3 min PI; 3 min. RBI	Rest	E: 135 min., with 3 x 10 min. CR; 6 min. RBI	Pool run E: 30 min.
8	Rest	E: 45 min., with two sets as 3 x 60 sec. OLP	Rest	E: 45 min., with 5 x 90 sec. FP; 60 sec. RBI	Rest	E: 90 min.	E: 30 min.

1 What it says: Rest.
What you do: Chill, sister.

2 What it says: Field test: E: 50 min. with 15 min. WU, 2 x 8 min. max efforts with 10 min. RBI
What you do: Put on a heart rate monitor. Spin easy, building to a moderate pace for 15 minutes. Then begin your field test: Take 45 seconds or so to build into the maximum effort you can hold for 8 minutes. Catch your breath for 10 minutes, then repeat. Record your average heart rate, and use the higher average heart rate to calculate your ranges. Cool down for 10 minutes.
More details: Your effort should be equivalent to a mile time trial at the track. Really push yourself, especially when you hit about 5 minutes down. And don't think about the second test while you're doing the first; your body will have plenty of time to recover.

3 What it says: E: 30 min., with OLP 2 sets of 3 x 30 sec.; 7 min. RBS
What you do: Warm up for about 10 minutes. Then take one foot out of a pedal (your feet should be secured to the pedal, either with cages on the pedals or clips on cycling shoes) and rest it on the bike frame so that it's out of the way. Pedal with one foot for 30 seconds. Then switch feet and pedal for 30 seconds. Repeat three times. Take 7 minutes at an endurance pace, then repeat the drill. Finish the ride at an endurance pace, gradually decreasing your effort.

4 What it says: E: 45 min., with 2 x 8 min. SS; 6 min. RBI
What you do: Warm up for about 10 minutes, then head into a steady-state interval (92 to 94 percent of your average max heart rate) for 8 minutes. Recover for 6 minutes, then repeat. Cool down with whatever time you have left.

5 What it says: E: 75–90 min., with 15 min. T
What you do: Ride in the endurance zone for 75 to 90 minutes. Somewhere in the middle, make your gear harder to reduce your cadence to 70 to 75 for a 15-minute tempo piece (tempo is 88 to 90 percent of your average max heart rate). When you're done, pop back up to an easier gear and finish your ride.
More details: Netflix or television helps on rides of more than 60 minutes. Just sayin'.

6 What it says: E: 45 min., with 5 x 60 sec. FP; 60 sec. RBI
What you do: Pedal in the endurance zone, and when you hit a spot where you want a little variety, make the gear a little easier and pedal as quickly as you can for 60 seconds. You shouldn't bounce in the saddle, though. Slow down those horses for 60 seconds; repeat five times total, then finish up the ride.

7 What it says: Pool run E: 30 min.
What you do: Head to chlorinated waters, jump in, and run in the deep end for 30 minutes. Your options are (not really) endless: You can either stay in one place or travel around the deep end, and you can use a belt or not (beginners might prefer one since a belt positions you properly).
More details: If you don't have—or can't stand—this option, you can ride endurance miles or, if your injury lets you, do the elliptical at the gym for the same amount of time.

8 What it says: E: 60 min., with two sets of 2 x 3 min. PI; 3 min. RBI; 10 min. RBS
What you do: In the course of a 60-minute endurance ride, crank up the intensity for a 3-minute power interval: You should be going all out, and your heart rate should be above your max average from your field test. Take 3 minutes to recover, then do another 3-minute piece. Pedal easy for 10 minutes, and repeat the whole shebang.
More details: Remember: You can do *anything* for 3 minutes. Or just about anything.

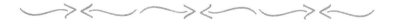

.1 TMI TUESDAYS: GREATEST HITS
By Sarah

As anyone who has ever run—or shared a hotel room—with me knows, I am Queen of Oversharing. It seemed only natural to me to carry this over to our Run Like a Mother: The Book Facebook page, so I started posting the occasional too-much-information status updates. Another mother runner named Erica suggested it become a weekly feature, dubbing it TMI Tuesday. A tradition—and a weekly highlight—was born. I culled a few posts and responses that made me laugh, snort, or even blush the most.

"Lawn care" question: Do running shorts and skirts (and swimsuits) make you feel more exposed, causing you to do more bush maintenance during these summer months? If so, what's your tool of choice—razor, Neet, waxing, other? Don't we all wish we could run as fast as the hair down there grows?

"My problem currently is trying to 'mow the lawn' blindly since I can't see past my 37-week belly. Terrifying adventure." —KENDRA

"How short are your skirts?" —LORRAINE

"Project BUSH, my favorite topic. Laser is the way to go. It's permanent and worth it. If you've given birth, laser is nothing." —KELLY

"I'm definitely a fan of waxing. For a hairy Italian like myself, there really is no better way to manage my forest. The process can be a bit like torture, but I pump on Advil beforehand." —NICOLE

"I will be looking over all of these responses. My razor makes me look worse than if I had just left it looking like a 1970s porno." —ALECIA

On our survey for *Train Like a Mother*, one gal said she skips sex the night before a race to avoid "drippage" during a race (ewww, but true). Anybody else say no to night-before nookie?

"Somehow reading this post makes me think of the song 'Smells Like Teen Spirit.' Ha, ha, ha." —JENNIFER

"Are you kidding? I've been married for almost 18 years. I take it whenever I can get it." —HEATHER

"Yikes! Maybe I shouldn't be eating breakfast while reading TMI Tuesday!" —EMILY

"Absolutely: I can't risk throwing my hip out!" —JENNIFER

"After having two babies, half the time I'm leaking with every footfall, anyway, so what's the difference?" —JENNIFER

"If I want to avoid hearing my husband bitch about having the kids all day while I run, then I had better go ahead and give it up." —ALECIA

"Agreed: No sex the night before a race, but two nights before, it's my go-to-sleep aid." —GINNY

"Girlfriend, lay off the Mucinex!" —STEPHANIE

This truly TMI question came to us via e-mail from a first-time half-marathoner who, post-race, has chafing of the butt crack. Eeek: Get that woman some Butt Paste or Desitin, stat! But the sufferer isn't looking for a solution, merely solidarity. Please assure her she's not alone. Anyone, anyone?

"I have a . . . uh . . . . . . friend that this happened to . . . yeah, a friend." —ANNE

"Oh, yeah, especially in the summer when all the sweat drips down and the cheeks rub together. Lovely! 2toms SportShield is my savior." —LESLIE

"BodyGlide your crack!" —JUANA

"OMG! This is utterly new to me! What a visual! Glad she is not alone. Can you imagine if you posted this . . . and nothing? Just the sound of cyber crickets chirping. Glad that didn't happen." —KRIS

"I have a separate BodyGlide just for that area." —AMY (NOTE: AMY LATER POSTED A PHOTO OF HER SPECIAL-USE-ONLY BODYGLIDE, CLEARLY LABELED "ASS.")

Toot, toot, it's TMI Tuesday. Here's the scene: SBS was recently running with a pal who shall remain nameless. She must have had a burrito or beans for din-din, as she was jet-propelled by gas that morning. SBS and the friend stayed mum whenever a gaseous emission was sounded, as if nothing had happened. What do you do when you pass gas while running with a friend, or when your friend toots?

"One of my running friends says, 'I think I just stepped on a duck,' and keeps running." —TERRY

"Definitely make a joke to lighten it up: Accuse her of having an unfair advantage." —DONNA

"Awkward. That's why I run alone." —AMELIA

"Although air may be passed, not a word is." —HEIDI

"We like to comment on the infestation of barking spiders." —KOURTNEY

"I giggle and tell my pards to stay upwind for their own safety." —E MMA

"Oh my, I am laughing so hard at some of the comments that I farted." —MARIANNE

11

NUTRITION: **EAT WELL TO RUN WELL**

By Dimity

On a random summer Thursday morning at 6 A.M., I grab a banana, my usual pre-workout fare, before heading to the neighborhood pool for a swim. The workout is intense—lots of short, fast laps—and I sip water, laced with fruit punch–flavored Nuun, when I stand in the shallow end to catch my breath. I arrive home about an hour later and down a glass of chocolate milk. Ever since I learned that *chocolate con leche* has been scientifically proven to have a nearly perfect recovery ratio of carbs to protein (3ish to 1), it's bookended nearly every workout of mine.

Then I walk over to the fridge to start my real breakfast, which always begins with a DIY latte made with skim milk and Oregon Chai, followed by a bagel or English muffin with some kind of nut butter. As I pop an English muffin in the toaster and the latte into the microwave, Ben saunters into the kitchen, smelling like a Porta-Potty. His pajama bottoms are soaked, so his sheets must be, too. I head upstairs to grab them and wash them.

I take out the latte and enjoy a sip before the whirlwind begins: a shower for me, a braid in Amelia's hair, a trip to the laundry room, some quick folding of towels, and a bunch of other tasks so trivial I can't recall them. An hour later, I spy the muffin, still in the toaster but now as stiff as cardboard. Not one to waste food, I slather some almond butter on it, microwave the honey bear so the last bit of crystallized honey will come out, drip golden drops onto the muffin, and cough the whole thing down with my cold latte. As I load the dishwasher, I finish the rest of Ben's banana and Amelia's remaining bite of pancake.

Not surprisingly, by 10:00, I'm famished. What I should eat to tide me over to lunchtime: yogurt, an apple, and a handful of almonds (all three things, not one of the above). But I'm instant-gratification hungry, so I opt for a generous handful of red-licorice nibs instead, and head back to the keyboard. In addition to the nibs sending me into an instant frenzy—I can almost feel the sugar buzzing in my brain—they are far from filling or satisfying. I trot back to the kitchen 10 minutes later for another overflowing handful, and then, 20 minutes later, I force myself to slowly step away from the nibs and grab two stalks of string cheese and a handful of Wheat Thins. An hour later, it's a chocolate chip Lärabar. On my way to Pilates at 2:30, I walk out the door with a handful, or three, of tortilla chips. Post-Pilates, I finally eat that apple, which I'd like to have with peanut butter, but slicing the apple, dealing with the peanut butter lid, and getting a plate feels like too much effort.

At 6:00 P.M. I am, once again, back at the pool—this time on the deck—and, once again, am ravenous. This time, I'm with both kids, and this time, I'd kill for a nib: I have nothing—not even a half of a box of stale raisins—in the pool bag. "Just one more jump," Amelia calls from the diving board, repeating a request I've assented to three times already. "Mom, judge my jump," says Ben, speed walking toward the board. If she went again, he reasons, he gets another go, too. Three more jumps later, I finally break the cycle, and they both grab their towels. "Hurry up," I tell them. "I'm starving."

If my kids were edible, I'd chomp on one of their arms.

On the way home, I make the executive decision to have grilled cheese for dinner: quick, easy, melted cheese. Makes us all happy. I unload the pool bag, let out the dogs, and hear a fight break out among the offspring. Pre-pool, we went to Walgreens for sunscreen, and I let them both pick out a cheap summer toy, which was mighty generous of me, seeing that I'd splurged on secondhand bikes and bulletin boards for both of them earlier in the week. Ben opted for a squirt gun and Amelia, a giant bubble wand. At the pool, the squirt gun was *the* toy to have, but now that we're on terra firma, the bubbles look much better, especially because there's only one wand, and Amelia isn't sharing. "I wanted bubbles, Mom! Why didn't you let me get bubbles?" Ben sobs and then screams, "I don't want a squirt gun! I want bubbles! I hate my squirt gun! Can we return it and get bubbles?"

I know he's 5, an age when the ability to have streamlined, rational thought, let alone understand the value of a dollar, is still in the oven, but my low-blood-sugared self is thinking like a 5-year-old, too. "Shut up! Just shut up!" I boom, and both my volume and my words surprise us all. I outlawed that phrase in our house, and I'm pretty sure I've never said—let alone yelled—it to my kids before. Amelia's eyes brim with tears. "I just bought you a bike this weekend, then I got you a bulletin board for your room, then a squirt gun, and now you're whining and crying over a two-dollar bubble wand! I can't handle this right now!" I continue yelling. "Go to your room until I say you can come out!"

Not surprisingly, they both dash from the kitchen. I'm beyond angry at myself, both for going nutso on my offspring and for thinking I could get through a typical workout/work/deal with kids/

errands day on snacks alone. I take a deep breath and slice cheese: One slice for the sandwiches, one hunk straight to my mouth. In less than 2 minutes, I have consumed a block of cheese about as big as Amelia's size-6 foot. I feel the crazies go away.

Even though I wasn't running a marathon, I hit the wall. Actually, I slammed into that sucker like I was at mile 20 of 26.2, and my kids paid the price. (I apologized to them for my behavior over our grilled cheeses—and used the opportunity for a little lesson about the importance of good nutrition.)

They aren't the only ones who take the hit, though. My 8-mile run the next day is less than pleasant: After about 4 miles, my legs get heavier and more lethargic. No amount of Espresso GU can perk them up. I drag my butt—now sorry in more ways than one—home.

TAKE IT *From* A MOTHER
WHAT'S YOUR FAVORITE SMOOTHIE RECIPE?

"I always eat this after a hard run or race: ½ cup of skim milk, ½ cup of egg whites, 1 banana, 2 teaspoons of peanut butter, 1 scoop of chocolate protein powder, and probably 1 teaspoon to 1½ teaspoons of wheat germ. If I don't have wheat germ, I use the same amount of crushed flax seeds."
—AMY (Dream running locale: "Not picky: just cool ocean breezes and flat terrain.")

"I thought 'yuck' when I found a recipe in Runner's World *for a kiwi, banana, and spinach smoothie. But I needed the iron and the protein, so I tried it. It is so good."*
—BETSY (Recipe from *Runner's World:* ½ cup of unsweetened almond milk; 1 cup of fresh spinach; 1 kiwi; sliced ½ banana, preferably frozen.)

"Here's an easy one that makes two servings: one for you, one for your running buddy. Or kid. 1 cup of fresh or frozen strawberries; 1 fresh or frozen banana, peeled; ½ cup of low-fat vanilla yogurt; ¾ cup of orange juice."
—TARA (Check out more of her recipes in her book *Almost Meatless: Recipes That Are Better for Your Health and the Planet*)

"I make smoothies with espresso powder, chocolate milk, frozen banana, and Greek yogurt."
—LISA (Favorite podcast on runs: *Stuff You Missed in History Class.*)

"I love my recovery smoothie: vanilla protein powder, frozen blueberries, milk, frozen mangos, frozen strawberries, and sugar-free chocolate pudding. Kiwis, if I have them."

—MARCI (TMI moment: Got a little number two—not hers—on the back of her leg in a Porta-Potty during a race. "Still makes me gag.")

"I love green smoothies. Stuff a blender with spinach and top it with banana, blueberries, water, and a scoop of whey protein powder."

—MEGAN (A gift for the 2005 Boston Marathon—light blue shorts and a matching top—went unused because Aunt Flo arrived race morning. She opted for black shorts, instead. "I don't wear the outfit much, but I think about it all the time.")

"My day is made by my morning smoothie: Knudsen Pineapple Coconut juice, vanilla Greek yogurt, shredded coconut, vanilla whey protein powder, old-fashioned oats, a splash of milk, one banana, frozen pineapple tidbits, frozen mango chunks, and spinach. Don't gag: The spinach makes all the difference in consistency and flavor—yum!"

—SBS (Hangs her sweaty workout wear on the back of her closet door and lets it air-dry rather than washing it after every run.)

At nearly 6 feet 4 inches, I am fortunate enough to have plenty of real estate over which to spread the nibs, the beers, the nachos, and the like, but that doesn't mean I don't have issues with food. (I've got lots of issues, actually, but I'll just focus on the nutrition-related ones here.) These days, as I work too hard and plan too little, my problems include no forethought (It's 5:30, and I have no plan for dinner. Life cereal, anybody?); way too much sugar (my instant pick-me-up when everything else feels too complicated); deceiving myself that I can eat well on the fly (How many granola bars and packs of Pretzel M&M's have I eaten over a steering wheel?); and generally relying too much on packaged meals and melted cheese for aforementioned unplanned dinners (quesadillas, grilled cheese, pizza). I don't particularly like to cook, either; any recipe requiring me to chop more than three things is usually a nonstarter. When I do don the oven mitts, it's usually to drain pasta to be paired with jarred sauce or for broiled chicken breasts.

I'm no Michael Pollan or Skinny Bitch, but I have given some thought to nutrition after that embarrassing blowup. Here are, in my mind, the dozen most important food rules for mother runners:

1. You must eat. We know you must run, so you must eat to have energy to go on sanity-saving runs. Many women run because they want to model healthy behavior for their children, yet then they distort the message when it comes to nourishing themselves. Feel free to count your calories, if need be, and be mindful of your food choices, but you must eat.

   In case my example of blowing up at my kids isn't instructional enough, realize there is a direct relationship between your level of hunger and the intelligence of choices you make. Starving? Everything looks good, especially Doritos, Hershey's Kisses, and leftover birthday cake. But if your stomach is just starting to speak up, carrots and hummus sound good, as does an orange or leftover salad.

2. You must eat relatively well. By relatively, I mean about 80 percent of the time. Eight out of 10 times, pick whole wheat over white. Fish over burgers. Fruit over chips. Hummus over ranch dressing. Grilled over fried. Sweet potato over french fries. Olive oil over butter. Low-fat over whole milk. Sorbet instead of ice cream.

   Don't drink your calories; eat a variety of colors; cook for yourself; be able to pronounce the ingredients you're ingesting; limit your purchases of food with packaging that proclaims, in neon letters, "All natural!"; use a bowl and a spoon—not just the latter—when you treat yourself to ice cream.

   Even when I heed most of these rules, I still fall into the mother trap: Feed my kids well, feed myself whatever. I cut up strawberries for their lunches, but go without fruit at my mid-day meal. I make sure they have veggies at least twice a day, but I cram in my (missed) daily quotient with a veggie-packed salad every second day or so. I give them milk with their meals, but drink a Diet Pepsi or glass of wine with mine.

   Still, I'm on track 80 percent of the time. At least when I'm not totally PMSing.

3. Set up your daily menu with a workout. Eating well and running are good bedmates; or, the more I run, the better I want to eat. Craptastic days like the above notwithstanding—there's an exception to every rule—there is definitely a correlation between how much I sweat out of my body and what I want to put into my body. On days I arrive home at 7:00 A.M., having already got my sweat on, I'm much less likely to think eight Thin Mints make a fine lunch and instead make a PB&J on whole wheat, eating it along with a clementine, a handful of cherry tomatoes, and two Thin Mints. (Okay, three.)

4. Know that running doesn't give you a pass to the all-you-can-eat buffet. Although I am very familiar with the I-just-ran-a-half-marathon-so-now-I-get-to-be-intimate-with-*both*-Ben-and-Jerry thought process, I also know the rationale is a little whack. *I'm going to do this really healthy thing, just so I can put a bunch of unhealthy food into my body.* Where's the logic in that?

Yes, running is definitely one of the best calorie torchers going—a good estimate is about 100 calories a mile—because it's so freakin' hard, but runners can still have high cholesterol, high blood pressure, and other health issues, especially as we age. Obviously, if you're so inclined, grab a burger, fries, and beer (or two) for a post-marathon dinner, and 2 hours later, eat a double scoop of mint chocolate chip ice cream. You've earned it. But every long run is not an excuse to eat a sleeve of Oreos.

The flip side of this thinking is equally as bunk: *I just burned 600 calories, so I'm going to maximize that by hardly eating anything today.* I get the lose-the-baby-weight thing, and I understand feeling terrible about your body when, after a winter of hibernation, your shorts are hugging your thighs too closely for comfort. Believe me: I study my butt in the mirror, lift it, and pretend I could lop off an inch of it. But then I move on—or get interrupted by Ben, who can't button his shorts—and try to remember that my generous glutes are actually my engines that get me up hills.

I'm not saying you can't lose weight and run at the same time, but do me—and the rest of womankind—a favor and focus on your performance, on the strength of your legs, and on the just-finished-a-run feeling instead of the random number on the label of your jeans. Last I checked, they don't mention your weight at your funeral (or put it on your headstone). But they will mention your love of running, your indomitable spirit, and your inspirational lifestyle.

5. Make carbs your friend. Despite the recent preponderance of bacon chocolate, bacon brownies, and bacon ice cream, pork—and any other form of protein—does not fuel a run. Carbs do. We'll keep the explanation *Sesame Street* simple: When you eat carbs, your body converts them to glycogen and stores them mostly in your muscles and liver. Glycogen is the gas you need to go the miles you want to. This doesn't mean an extra-large helping of penne every night, but don't fall into the Paleo, South Beach, or diet du jour trap.

6. Figure out your pre-run plan. Some people need to have something in their stomach before a run, while others can't tolerate it. You'll know fairly quickly into which camp you fall.

If your run is less than an hour, you can get away with simply going, although I prefer, as you know, a banana in my stomach. Longer than that, and I need a lighter meal. Typically,

I eat something bland about an hour before a long run: could be banana and peanut butter on an English muffin; a small bowl of oatmeal with brown sugar and raisins; yogurt and a piece of toast; whatever sounds good. Smoothies (see recipes on 167) are a good option if your stomach rejects solid food. If I'm racing, I extend that window to 2 hours; I want to have things pretty well digested, as well as all the, um, waste removed from my system before I get to the starting line.

The key with this whole scenario is to make it superfamiliar and easy for you to handle. Before every long run on Saturday while training for the half-marathon, you have two pieces of multigrain toast with butter and jam. Guess what you'll eat before the race? One less thing to worry about.

7. Plan an on-the-run plan. For runs longer than 90 minutes, you need fuel; as strong and capable as your muscles are, they run out of glycogen around then. Your body takes to burning your fat stores on runs longer than 90 minutes—and who doesn't like the sound of that?—but it takes two to tango: Fat needs glycogen in order to metabolize. (Personally, I carry a gel on runs longer than an hour, because I never know when the hungries might strike. Plus, I'll take any excuse to stop for a minute or two.)

As with your breakfast, do your own experimentation to determine what you'll stuff in the doll-size pockets on most running gear. It sounds like a bit of a cop-out, but what works for my nearly bombproof stomach can wreak havoc on your delicate innards. What I can tell you: Nearly anything that has simple, easy-to-digest sugar can work for fuel. Try gummi bears, Tootsie Rolls, raisins, your kids' fruit snacks, malted milk balls (be careful of the melting), and anything you can buy at your local running store in silvery packets for what feels like steep prices. (Again, no Muscle Builder Extra Wow Mega Protein Bars: Protein is for after, not during, the run.)

8. Don't let your stomach throw a tantrum. Nancy Clark, a goddess of sports nutrition, reports the following:

• Women have more gastrointestinal (GI) issues than men, especially when we're on the rag. ("The hormonal shifts that occur during menstruation can contribute to looser bowel movements," she explains in her *Sports Nutrition Guidebook*.)

• Runners, who are basically jumping from one foot to the other, have more GI issues than cyclists, swimmers, and other athletes who maintain a more stable position.

• Beginning runners have more GI issues than more experienced athletes because their poop

PRACTICAL *Motherly* ADVICE
CRUNCHING NUMBERS

Break out the calculator; it's time for some math. Promise, we won't ask you what the Pythagorean theorem[1] is. Instead, here are some strategies to help you nail your nutrition.

For runs longer than 90 minutes: Take in between 200 and 300 calories per hour, or 50 to 75 grams of carbs per hour. Begin your fueling before you hit 90 minutes, so that you don't empty the tank then have to refill from empty. I like to take in a gel about 30 minutes into a long run. Definitely get some calories into you before you hit 45 minutes, so that you don't deplete your glycogen stores prematurely.

Some ideas:

One packet of GU: 25 grams of carbs, 100 calories

3 Clif Shot Bloks: 25 grams of carbs, 100 calories

10 gummi bears: 23 grams of carbs, 87 calories

2 tablespoons of raisins: 22 grams of carbs, 91 calories

12 Dots: 35 grams of carbs, 140 calories

8 ounces of Gatorade: 14 grams of carbs, 50 calories

For recovery from any run longer than 60 minutes or an intense run, such as speedwork, intervals, or a tempo run: First, massage a few numbers to figure out how many grams of carbs and protein you need to get in your bod, post-run:

1. Multiply your weight in pounds by .3 to get the amount of carbs in grams.
2. Pretend I weigh 140 pounds (I did, probably, in ninth grade. Too bad I wasn't a runner then.) 140 pounds x .3 = 42 grams of carbs for recovery
3. Then you want a 3:1 carbs-to-protein ratio to optimize both replenishing your glycogen and your muscle recovery. So, take 42 grams, divide that by 3 to figure out your protein needs. 42/3 = 14 grams
4. Within 30 minutes, the optimal time to hit the "gas station," you'd want to consume something like:
   - 12 ounces of chocolate milk (40 g of carbs, 11 g of protein)
   - 1 bagel and 2 tablespoons of peanut butter (45 g of carbs, 9 g protein)
   - Egg-white omelet, veggies, and a plate of fruit, with a side of whole-wheat toast (about 35 g of carbs, 12 g of protein)

---

[1] If you can't recall, it's $a^2 + b^2 = c^2$. Applies to triangles.

- 1 cup of Greek yogurt and fruit (30 g of carbs, 11 g of protein)
- Vivanno protein shake from Starbucks (50 g of carbs, 18 g of protein)

For the rest of the day, keeping the same carbs-to-protein ratio isn't a bad idea, as you'll continue to restock your glycogen and encourage the rebuilding of muscle.

For carbo-loading: Carbo-loading, which is what you need to do for marathons and half-marathons, is an insidery way of saying topping off your tank, so that you have as much easy-to-access fuel as possible in your body on race day. Basically, you want to switch most of your calorie intake to carbs 2 to 3 days before you go the distance. Again, pretend I'm a svelte 140 pounds and play along.

1. Divide your current weight in pounds by 2.2 to get kilograms. 140/2.2 = 63.6 kilograms

2. Multiply the number of kilograms by 8 to get the amount of carbs you need to eat on Friday and Saturday for a marathon or half-marathon on Sunday. 63.6 x 8 = 509 grams of carbs

3. Now pull your calculator and scale, head to the pantry, and count out exactly 509 grams . . . wait, can't swing it?

Here's an example of a hefty, hearty day of carbo-loading. Enjoy—you've worked hard for it!

Breakfast
A 4-inch bagel: 50 grams
2 tablespoons strawberry jam: 26 grams
1 medium banana: 27 grams
8 ounces low-fat, yogurt: 35 grams
8 ounces orange juice: 25 grams
Total: 163 grams

Snack
Nature Valley Oats 'n' Honey Granola Bar
   (2 bars): 29 grams
8 ounces Gatorade: 14 grams
Total: 43 grams

Lunch
½ package prepared Kraft Macaroni &
   Cheese: 50 grams[1]
1 sourdough roll: 40 grams
8 ounces chocolate milk: 25 grams
Total: 115 grams

_____

[1] I'm assuming you're eating with the kids.

Snack
2 slices white bread: 25 grams
2 tablespoons strawberry jam: 26 grams
8 ounces Gatorade: 14 grams
Total: 65 grams

Dinner
A chicken burrito at Chipotle with 4 ounces
of black beans, 3 ounces of rice, 3.5 ounces
of corn salsa: 105 grams (add guacamole for 8
more grams)
A 12-ounce beer: 13 grams
Total: 126 grams (w/guac)

GRAND TOTAL: 512 GRAMS

Note: If you feel the need to jump on the scale during the carbo-loading, tapering phase, be prepared to see the needle zing up anywhere from 2 to 4 pounds from your normal weight. Don't freak—and definitely don't go for a long run to burn it off. The extra weight means you get a gold star for carbo-loading; every ounce of stored carbs comes with an add-on gift: about 3 ounces of water. So you've basically gained water weight, and you'll sweat it off over 13.1 or 26.2 miles. I promise.

chutes take time to get adjusted to all the jostling, and their bodies haven't been primed to drop a deuce on command.

- Harder workouts—anything where you're going beyond a conversational pace—produce more GI issues than easy ones.

- Dehydration, high-fiber diets, and too much coffee or sugar can also hit the GI.

Needless to say, her warnings don't bode well for a new female runner who has to have caffeine, is having her period, and is headed out to do some intervals. Keep the intestines as quiet as possible by heeding the same advice for training properly: Don't start out running too hard, too fast, or too long, and let your body adjust to running. A couple of mother runners we've heard from swear by taking Imodium to keep things firm; if you want to go that route, definitely try it on a training run when you can loop near home or your car in case matters get urgent.

9. Think about the drink. Heed this commonsense advice from Ilana Katz, a knowledgeable, realistic sports nutritionist and Ironman triathlete:

- Two hours pre-run, drink 8 to 16 ounces of fluid.[1] Fluid can mean either water or an enhanced drink, such as Nuun or Gatorade.

- 15 to 30 minutes before you head out, chug 4 to 8 ounces of fluid.

- During a run longer than 60 minutes, drink 4 to 8 ounces every 15 to 20 minutes.

---

[1] If you're running at 5:30 A.M., obviously don't wake up at 3:30 to drink. But if you're up at 5:30 to head to a race that starts at 8:00, drink up.

- Post-run, the best way to know how much to drink is to complete a little DIY science experiment, which Katz recommends:

    a. On a day with typical temperatures when you run, weigh yourself naked before you head out.
    b. Get dressed and run for 60 minutes. Don't pee or drink during, or immediately after, this run.
    c. Strip, and weigh yourself again.
    d. For every pound you lost, replace with 16 to 24 ounces of fluid. Erring on the higher side is a little like lowering a basketball hoop for a 7-year-old: There's a better chance of hitting the target.

    The beauty of this sweat-rate experiment? Now you know more specifically how much you need to drink during a longer run. Say you lost 1.5 pounds during that 60-minute run. 1.5 x 16 ounces = 24 ounces. If you're running for 2 hours, aim to drink 48 ounces (2 x 24 ounces) to keep yourself hydrated during the run, instead of becoming dehydrated and then having to replenish your stores after your workout.

10. **Cook with leftovers in mind.** When I get motivated to make a decent dinner, I always make more than I should. I cook 2 cups of brown rice instead of one; double a recipe for veggie chili; make lasagne and freeze half of it. When I make a salad, I don't dress it, so that we can eat it the following lunch or dinner. Yes, by Thursday, I'm certainly sick of the pasta/spinach/chick pea/olive oil combo thing I made for dinner on Monday, but at least I know it's good food.

    SBS is good at giving new life to leftovers for lunchtime salads: Her orzo with pine nuts side dish is satisfying when it's served cold with the inclusion of cherry tomatoes, chopped feta, chopped green onions, and some vinaigrette dressing. Lentils can get tossed with red onion, arugula, feta—which is always on hand in her fridge—and an easy mustard–olive oil dressing.

11. **Don't expect to lose crazy amounts of weight through serious training.** When you go from a sedentary lifestyle to all gaga over running, your body will obviously get on board, and shed pounds upon pounds in its quest to become a runner. I've read countless tales of losing 30, 50, 75 pounds through running. Love those stories. But many women equate running more with losing more, and that isn't the case, as I've also heard again and again. Once your body gets used to running and "levels out," the pounds don't just melt off with mileage. Intense training oftentimes makes you *gain* weight. It is the good, heavier, muscle weight, and it's likely you look even more kick-

ass in your tall boots and short skirt, but the scale won't reflect it. And, it should be noted, if you are training intensely, you need to feed your body. (See rule 1.)

12. Try not to buy junk. Easier said than done, I realize. But there's a reason why I "borrow" my kids' leftover Halloween candy when I'm having a bout of writer's block, PMS, or a fit of pissiness at my husband. It's the only junk food in the house. I've bought too many 1-pound bags of M&M's ("They're on sale," I reason with my drooling self, "and I'll add them to GORP.") only to have them gone within days.

When I simply can't live without a Kit Kat/scoop of Nutella/cupcake and have none in the house, I have to go out and get it. When I think about the task of piling two kids in the car and explaining the treat is for me, not them, suddenly that craving doesn't seem as overwhelming as it used to. (Or I can at least wait and have my husband pick it up on his way home from the office.)

One other strategy I use: buying a small amount—20 yogurt-covered pretzels or a scoop of gumdrops—in the bulk aisle. Do not misread: not *in* bulk. Nothing good can come of the candies, cookies, and other sugar-laden snacks they offer at Costco. I made that mistake once, and 8,000 calories of chocolate-covered almonds later, I don't think I'll ever eat another one. (They're on my can't-tolerate-anymore list, along with Jägermeister and double-cheese pizza from Pizza Hut.)

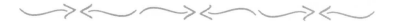

.1 THE RUNNING PATH[1]
By Dimity (kind of)

Once there was a running path and she loved a young mother runner. And every day—or as many days as she could make it—the mother runner would run on her dirt and next to her trees and play queen of the world. She would climb her hills and cruise on the flats and eat a GU. And when she was running downhill, she pretended she could always run that fast. And when she was tired, she would stretch in the shade of the path. The mother runner loved the path very much. And the path was happy.

But time went by. And the mother runner got faster. And wanted to run longer. And the path was often alone. Then one day, on another run, the mother runner ran by the path and the path said, "Come, mother runner, come climb up and fly down my hills and eat a GU. Run and be happy."

"I am beyond your 2-mile length. I am training for a 10K," said the mother runner. "My training plan has me running for 5 miles today. I need distance. Can you give me distance?"

"I'm sorry," said the path, "but I can't grow. I have only hills and shade. But run my hills, mother runner, again and again, and you will be strong and you will go fast." So the mother runner ran up the hills again and again, and she became fast. And the path was happy.

But the mother runner stayed away for a long time and the path was sad. And then one day the mother runner came back. The path shook with joy and she said, "Come, mother runner, climb up and fly down my hills and cruise through my shade and be happy."

"I am too busy to cruise. I am training for a half-marathon," said the mother runner. "I want a vacation with my girlfriends and a chance to sleep in a quiet hotel room and a plane ride with nobody but me eating my Swedish fish, and so I need to run a half-marathon. Can you help me?"

"I am only 2 miles long," said the path, "but my shade is plenty. Come finish your long runs in my shade and I will make sure your last miles are pleasant." So the mother runner finished her long runs in the cool shade. And the path was happy.

But the mother runner stayed away for a long time. And when she came back, the path was so happy she could hardly speak. "Come, mother runner," she whispered. "Come and run."

"I am too sad to run," said the mother runner. "I am injured from doing too many races and am not sure I'll ever run again. Right now, I just want to run far away. Can you help me?"

"Start here and walk," said the path. "Then you can heal and run again and be happy." And so the mother runner started to walk on the path, and then she got healthy and ran many more miles. And the path was

---

[1]Inspired by *The Giving Tree* by Shel Silverstein, a children's classic that never fails to make both SBS and me simultaneously smile and tear up.

happy. But not really.

And after a long time the mom came back again. "I am sorry, mother runner," said the path, "but I have nothing left for you. My hills aren't steep enough for you."

"My quads are too weak for big hills," said the mother runner.

"Some trees have died and my shade isn't as deep as it used to be," said the path. "You can't cruise through it."

"I can hardly cruise anymore," said the mother runner.

"At least you can still come and eat GU on me," said the path.

"My stomach can't stomach GU anymore," said the mother runner.

"I am sorry," sighed the path. "I wish that I could give you something, but I have nothing left. I am just an old path."

"I don't need very much now," said the mother runner. " I don't need to run fast or far anymore. I just need a quiet place to run and find my spirit. I simply want to run."

"Well," said the path, straightening herself up as much as she could, "Well, an old path is good for just running. Come, mother runner, run. Run and smile." And the mother runner did. And the path—and the mother runner—were happy.

12

RACE GOALS: **EYEING THE RIGHT PRIZE**

By Sarah

The unrelenting California sun, reflected off the pavement and sneaking behind my Oakley shades, makes me squint. When I turn my head to take in the beauty of the blooming mustard and curlicue grapevines—this is the Napa Valley Marathon, after all—all I see are sunspots. The supposedly flat point-to-point course had served up some longish climbs that sure felt like hills, especially after I went out too fast, hitting the half-marathon mark in a who-knew-I-could-do-it 1:53. My last roadside meet-up with Jack and 14-month-old Phoebe feels like it was yesterday, not 45 minutes ago.

Fortunately, I'm not alone. My good friend Stacy W. (aka SW) jumped into the race near mile 19 to run with me to the finish of this, my third, marathon, just as she did for me in the San Francisco and New York City marathons. And as in marathons one and two, after running with her for a few miles, I start to backpedal on my goal of breaking 4 hours. "Forget it, SW," I tell her, going on a rant that's in rhythm with my footsteps. "Trying to break 4 hours is stupid. I was a moron for thinking I could do it. My legs are killing me. I don't care anymore. I just want to finish. For real, I don't care if I break 4 hours. Really." SW, a veteran of several 26.2-mile races, knows hitting the wall—feeling lead-legged, nauseated, and totally tapped out—can mess with a runner's resolve, and I'm no exception. When we hit the 23-mile marker, she reminds me how I'd wanted to break 4 hours before, and been supremely disappointed at coming up short. She points out I missed my goal in San Francisco by mere minutes. She says I'm strong. She says I am looking good. (Liar!) She tells me I can do it.

I tell her she's wrong. I inform her I'm not sure I can make it to the finish line, or even the next mile marker. "Marathons suck hard," I tell her, spiraling down into a hole no forklift could pull me out of. "It's stupid to run this far." (For the record, I possess an extensive vocabulary, but after mile 20 of most marathons, "stupid," "suck," and several Parental Advisory words dominate my

178

lingo.) I tell her, once again, I don't give a s@#t about any goals I set out before the race.

That was then, this is now. And now, to quote myself, sucks hard.

I've run four more marathons since that spectacular, but typical, downfall, and my running has changed quite a bit since then. For my debut 26.2, as you know, I made up my workouts as I went along. For Rounds 2 and 3, I used training plans that were super-basic and didn't include the intensity my body needed to see a sub-4-hour finish. I mistakenly thought I could get to 3:59 with merely a decent level of cardiovascular fitness, a mighty dose of adrenaline, SW by my side for the later miles, and an unfounded optimism I could fly through the race like I'd never done in training. What I almost always forgot was that pain and exhaustion catch up with me, and steal all the wind out of my running skirt, and leave me despondent, desperate, drained, and every other negative adjective beginning with "d." (Dazed. Delusional. Dejected. Distressed. *Dead.*)

Now, thanks to endless loops around the local track, I can run faster. But even doing 6 x 800 meters more times than I can remember doesn't guarantee I won't lose my drive on race day—or in the days leading up to the start line. Take my most recent 26.2, the 2010 Portland Marathon, which was in October (I had run Big Sur—see chapter 1—in April of that same busy year). Even though this was my second time through it that year, I still followed my fairly advanced training schedule to the letter. Throughout the first 11 weeks of the 12-week plan, I talked and blogged, and blogged and talked some more, about my two-pronged goal on race day: to qualify for Boston, which involved crossing the finish line in less than 4 hours, and to shave about 2½ minutes off my personal record and run under 3:50. Given my familiarity with the home course and my legs, which still felt strong from my diligent hill training for Big Sur, I thought I had a good shot at reaching both. Plus, come on: It would be cool to PR in my hometown with fam and friends cheering me on.

What solidified my more ambitious goal was that the training partner I had recently found to share long runs with, Sheila, also had the fire in her belly to finish faster than 3:50. Her PR was 59 seconds—no, not one full minute—faster than mine so we had both come close. We were a well-matched pair, fueling each other's dream as we racked up miles around Portland. Sheila, her husband, and their two sons, who were close in age to my brood, had recently moved to town from New York City by way of Vermont. A pharmacist with a warm personality and sly wit, Sheila was easygoing about our routes, letting me map out our courses.

One Saturday in mid-September, when it was a bit hotter than we would have liked, I ran the 2 miles to her house for the start of a 16-mile outing. We headed south toward Mount Tabor, an extinct volcano flanked by towering coniferous trees. As we loped down residential streets, our conversation easily moved from the DVD she'd watched the night before, to her husband's quest to open his own restaurant, to my twins' antics in the first few weeks of kindergarten.

Skirting the edge of Mount Tabor, we veered toward the Willamette River, which bisects the heart of the city. I drained the water bottles on my Amphipod, but we stopped for GU (me) and Clif Shot Bloks (Sheila) and cool slurps from ever-gurgling water fountains once we reached the waterfront. Fifteen minutes later, starting the slight climb from the river to my neighborhood, I started feeling overheated and slightly nauseated. We were 2 miles from my house, and my Garmin said I had covered almost 13 miles. (Sheila still had to run the additional 2 miles back to her house to complete her 16). I started daydreaming about running directly home, cutting my run short by roughly a mile. I silently clung to that notion for the next 10 minutes. As we got closer to my digs, I told Sheila my plan, saying I was running on reserves.

Run LIKE THIS MOTHER
EVERYBODY WINS!

By Dimity

These days, when kids get rewarded for everything from brushing their teeth to playing T-ball at recess, there's a chance we parents, teachers, and coaches may have taken the whole you-rock! thing a little too far. Reality will hit hard when they realize that, in fact, they don't get a blue participation ribbon for simply showing up to their job.

For us mother runners, however, there is no such thing as too much glory at a race's end. Many (blinder-wearing) runners will say the only worthy race goal is a time goal. While I respect that opinion, I don't believe it. Despite one's best intentions and preparation, races rarely go as planned. Weather blows in. Your quads blow up. Your intestines blow out—and hopefully into a Porta-Potty. If I've trained and focused on one race for 3 months, then I miss my one, lonely time goal, I'm not going to be in a good place, post-race. Speaking from experience, I know there will be too many tears and too much rumination, which isn't fair to me or my family, who supported me through my training. One race result does not define a training cycle—or me.

How do I avoid the finish-line drama? I embrace a we're-all-winners mentality by setting a variety of goals. Some naysayers may compare this to a fish/barrel/gun scenario, but to them, I say "Pshaw." According to Running USA, 13 million Americans crossed a finish line in 2010. Sounds like a lot until you consult the U.S. Census Bureau, which reports 308 million people reside in our fair land. Working the numbers, that means about 4.2 percent of all the people in the U.S. ran a race in 2010—and, don't quote me on this, but I bet the percentage is actually lower, seeing that most (addictive-personality) runners don't run only one 10K a year and call it good. So that's a long-winded way of saying: You get to feel accomplishment when you finish a race, no matter how dismal your race was.

Back to this multiple-goals thing. Some coaches and exceptionally driven people do set multiple goals, but they're usually both time goals, and they call them A and B goals. I like the sentiment, but how fulfilling does it feel to say, "I met my B goal"? It's like dry humping: It's fine, but you know you can get better. Instead, I prefer to describe my running goals as good, better, and best—and highly recommend you take a page out of my book (uh, not literally).[1]

GOOD GOALS

For me, these are time-oriented goals, like setting a PR, hitting certain splits, coming in under some finishing time, beating my husband (kidding, oh love of my life). I often vocalize one ambitious but achievable good goal, and keep at least one slower, but still acceptable, good goal in my head.

For instance, at a half-marathon, prior to which my longest training run was 11 miles at a pace that wouldn't get me to a sub-2-hour finish, I mentioned I wanted a sub-2:00 finish to anybody who asked. But I also branded 2:05 in my brain, knowing that was more realistic and a little generous, timewise. I finished in a satisfying 2:02, nicely meeting a good goal.

BETTER GOALS

These smaller goals aren't related to any strict numbers. Instead, they're about the place I am with my running story right now, and how I want this race chapter to play out.

Mental toughness is, and will always be, a huge hurdle for me, so one better goal might be to not walk when I really want to. Another better goal might be to check in with my form (Am I standing tall? Taking small steps? Relaxing my upper body?) regularly. I could also make one for running a smart race: making sure I don't go out too fast, eat when I should, drink enough fluids, and feel like I've given my all when I hit the end.

The beauty of better goals is that during the race I mentally shuffle through them, like songs on

---

[1] The beauty of having the three-tiered goal plan is the answer you have when somebody asks you about your race. If you've knocked it out of the park, gush all you like. But if the outcome wasn't quite as you'd had in mind, you can simply say, "I set some good goals, and I did even better than that." Or, "I had some pre-race goals, and I achieved my best one."

an iPod, stopping on the one that feels best at that moment. When I don't feel like being mentally tough, I allow myself to walk but am sure to eat a gel during my brief stroll. Lookie there: a better goal achieved!

BEST GOALS

I have my good and better goals, which rotate from race to race, set in my mind before the race starts, but the best goal is evergreen: simply to get across the line, no matter how I look or how long it takes me.

I pull out my best goal when I'm running a longer-distance race for the first time in years; when my stomach decides it's staging a rave; or when something out of my control—my menstrual cycle, a sudden injury, a killer course—is flipping me the bird. Then it's time to adjust my perspective and remember not to be overly concerned that my footsteps are louder than a bass drum, or that my splits are more depressing than the national debt. "I'm doing what only 4.2 percent of Americans have the motivation and courage to do," I tell myself. "That, in and of itself, makes me a rock star."

As I mentally will the next mile marker to show up .75 miles early, I have a hard time believing that bold statement at the time. But as soon as I cross the line, you can bet I feel the best I have in miles.

Sheila would hear none of it. "No, you've gone this far—don't conk out so close to the full distance. Come on." A mere three straight blocks from my house, she became the run leader, and made us turn right. She said we'd just go a bit east, zigzag up and down a few blocks, then head back west. "We don't need to go very far to add up to a mile—not even all the way to Grant High School." Grant, our neighborhood high school, seemed as far away as my twins are from attending it.

Sheila didn't have to drag me, but it was close at times. Finally the digits on my wrist told us we'd made up enough ground. Sheila peeled off toward her house, picking up her pace, while I nearly crawled the final one-sixth of a mile home.

I should have realized then Sheila had stronger resolve than I did.

Yet I was rock-solid resolute with the qualify-for-Boston *and* run sub-3:50 plan for about 80 days. Then, two-thirds of the way through the taper, something shifted. I broke loose of my mooring and felt adrift in my convictions. It wasn't physical; my body felt fine. Nothing hurt, nothing felt overused. But hesitation slowly seeped into my system. I'm not sure why, but I had a nagging sense my body—and my brain—weren't up for maximum effort. Maybe the memory of going the distance at Big Sur was too fresh in my mind. I *emptied* myself on that racecourse. Or perhaps my muscles, which had stayed strong and fresh through 24 weeks of intense training, led the charge. Maybe they were trying to tell me they didn't have PR firepower in them. Or it could be I was just too much of a wimp to embrace the effort I knew I'd need to summon at game time.

However my unwillingness got there, it was soon omnipresent. It circulated through my body until it reached my brain. My very capable and fit resolve dissolved like a Nuun tablet in a bottle of water. Every day, I could feel the uncertainty building in intensity, and my desire slipping away. What had seemed supremely important for months now seemed insignificant. Why did I need to BQ *and* PR? Certainly qualifying for Boston was more than good enough, right?

As soon as I let that Beantown-is-plenty thought be fully articulated in my head, it elbowed out my PR dream, which didn't stand a chance against that bully. Half of me, the fueled-by-bravado side, was disappointed at this new world order. I felt like I was wimping out, like I lacked the courage and grit other mother runners, like Sheila, have to push beyond self-perceived limits.

But my other more realistic half cut me some slack. In the days leading up to the race, I wasn't merely eating pasta, visualizing a 3:49 finish, and taking it easy. I was on Another Mother Runner duty, hawking our book and tees and chatting with the tribe at the race expo. (I love doing it, but it's not ideal the day before 26.2.) Plus, since the marathon was on my home turf, unlike all my other long races that required some travel, I still had to deal with everyday demands. Making school lunches, corralling the kids to bed, grocery shopping, doing laundry, and all the other wifely/motherly duties I don't need to list for you.

The days before the marathon, I still hadn't told Sheila my revised race plan. As she and I texted back and forth—Are you wearing arm warmers? Are you riding public transportation to the start line? Have you seen the weather forecast?—I kept wanting to actually call her. But to voice my decision would be to accept a small defeat before I even pinned on my race number. It was selfish, I know, to keep silent, but by that point, I was having trouble keeping my head in the game. Could I even BQ anymore? Hashing out race strategy with someone else, even Sheila, would have sent me spiraling.

Instead, I didn't speak up until the starting line.

Sheila and I—along with thousands of other Portland Marathoners—crowded together under office building awnings, trying to evade the raindrops falling fast and furious on the downtown streets. I turned to my devoted long-run partner, and said, "Any chance you want to run just sub-4? I'm thinking I won't go for under 3:50. Sub-4 is enough to get me to Boston." Just like that, any remnants of my willpower washed down a storm drain along with the rain and brown autumn leaves.

A confused, somewhat startled look flashed across Sheila's usually brightly smiling face. She shook her head, saying, "Uh-uh: I'm going to try to PR. Why would I change my mind now?" Somewhat disappointed I couldn't win her over to my wimpier ways, I envied her acceptance to embrace the challenge to the very end.

The way Sheila and I felt going into that marathon reminds me that race goals are, in some ways, like a sports bra or a pair of running shoes: What fits and feels great on your friend might chafe or be too heavy on you. I should know, as I've had goals that run from gasping from start to finish to laughing along the way. Admittedly, I am driven by time goals, but as you can now tell, I don't always stand firm on those convictions. My marathon goal that felt so right—and so brass-ring reachable—in July seemed like trying to touch the stars by early October.

Goal setting—and goal keeping—depends so much on what is going on in your life. Unless you're a pro athlete, where it's your *job* to prep and execute a race, the day-to-day always should play a role in determining what you want to accomplish in a given race. As much as we love it, running and racing add stress to our lives. If you don't consider the big picture, the stress can take on a life of its own and suck all the joy and pride out of training.

Say, for instance, your husband is deployed overseas 4 months before your half-marathon; suddenly you have to do most of your training on a treadmill after the kiddos go to sleep. Trying to set a personal record at that half is probably not the best idea. (Unless it's your *first* 13.1, then of course you'll PR!) The year your oldest starts high school, your middle child heads off to middle school, and your youngest is suddenly struggling with his fourth-grade teacher is not the ideal time to tackle 26.2 for the first time. Opt for a shorter race or two in the fall, and sign up for a spring marathon, instead. Returning to racing after an injury? Manage your personal expectations and contemplate "pacing not racing" the distance. And, suffice it to say, any race done within 6 months of having a baby is not the best to pin many goals on beyond finishing with a smile on your face and receiving a slobbery kiss after the race.

Once you've set your goals, they cling to your brain like your preschooler holds her lovey at bedtime. Then, on race day, when the sun beats down too hard, your iPod battery dies, your knee tweaks near mile 7, or you wake up with a simmering sinus infection, you can feel your goals shifting and sliding out of your grasp. It can be tough to know when to let go and when to hold on for dear life. Remember that everyone encounters doubts and rough spots in races. When stinking thinking arises, try banishing it by taking in some energy or fluid. Your brain might be trying to shut down your underfueled body. As you fill back up, tell yourself that a few minutes of "This hurts; I hate this!" is no reason to toss aside the dreams and aspirations you clutched tightly during training.

TAKE IT *From* A MOTHER
DO YOU CONSIDER YOURSELF MENTALLY TOUGH?

"Yes. I have multiple sclerosis, and sometimes this causes me to lose gains I have made. My muscles get weak, or my legs get spastic. When this happens, I have to start my training all over again. But I have found that each time I begin again, the recovery time to where I was is shorter because I continually get stronger, tougher, and more determined."
—DAWN (Favorite pre-run snack: a banana and a Hershey bar. Alternate bites between the two.)

"No. Not really. Fears prey on me disproportionate to reality. It's been a habit for so long that they're hard to shake, and that makes me feel weak."
—HOLLY (Gets lost in books on tape during runs.)

"Yes. I ran a marathon while passing kidney stones. I won't quit until I pass out, unless it's raining. Then I will go to Starbucks and call it a day."
—AMANDA (If she's running fewer than 20 miles a week, she's either "on vacation or nearly dead.")

"I'm working on it, but definitely not when I started running. I've got enough runs under my belt now to know I'm not really going to die."
—KATIE (Felt like a real runner when she had surgery and every nurse who took her heart rate asked, "Are you a runner?")

"My mental game is by far my weakest attribute as an endurance athlete. On good days, I'm unstoppable. But when my mental toughness gets a crack in it, I fall hard."
—TONIA (Owns eight pairs of compression socks. "That way, I can wear a pair every day if I want.")

"Yes. I've done two tours in Iraq, finished a marathon, and given birth in a tub in my living room."
—BETHANY (Favorite podcast to listen to while running: NPR's Wait Wait . . . Don't Tell Me!)

"Absolutely! Giving birth to eight children will do that to a woman. There have been times when I honestly felt I couldn't go another step, but dug down deep enough to suck it up and finish the run."
—CATEY (Refers to those suck-it-up moments as a conversation with her "inner Jillian Michaels.")

If a course ends up being dramatically different than what you trained for, modify your goals on the fly. This happened to me in the marathon Dimity and I ran in San Francisco. Yes, despite the host city, I didn't prep with enough hill training. (I know, I know. . . .) When I hit the halfway point in 2:02, I knew a better-than-4-hour marathon wasn't in my pocket that day. I wallowed in self-pity for a few miles, then told myself I was going to keep pushing, vowing to pass at least five runners each mile.

If the impediment is physical—a sudden injury or illness—let go of your goal and seek medical attention. Ashley, a badass mother runner who was also running the 2010 Portland Marathon, became severely disoriented and woozy near mile 25 of her first marathon. Luckily, her dad had jumped into the race to run the final miles with her; instead, he steered her toward the medical tent. It wasn't the marathon finish Ashley had imagined, but stopping meant she was well enough to qualify for the venerable Boston Marathon in her next 26.2-mile endeavor.

The rain was still falling hard around mile 15 of the Portland Marathon. Despite it being after 9 A.M., it was dark as dusk as I dodged streamlike puddles along a flat, desolate stretch of highway. Two miles before, the face of my Garmin had fogged up—on the inside. I could scarcely make out the elapsed time; forget about reading my pace. I was running naked (read: no time or pace, not sans clothes). For the rest of the race, I was basically clueless to how close I was to reaching either of my goals. Around mile 21, my good friend and two-time veteran of this marathon, Ellison, handed me a fresh bottle of water and a packet of blueberry–pomegranate Roctane gel. We exchanged only a few words, but I knew her well enough to pick up a sense of urgency in her encouragement to stay strong.

I ended up qualifying for Boston by the skin of my teeth. As in 65 seconds to spare. (Alas, Sheila missed both goals, finishing in 4:02.) Obviously, I'll never know what I could have achieved that day if I hadn't let go of my under-3:50 goal. Given the lousy weather and my Garmin malfunction, I don't regret not going for it. The speedier finish time felt like too onerous of a task, and I needed to throw it aside to let me reach my "easier" goal.

One thing I *do* know: By having a Plan B in place, I was able to savor my Boston-qualifying time instead of lamenting my missed A goal. Qualifying for Boston wasn't a gimme, but it was more firmly in my grasp. My marathon pal SW wasn't by my side that day, but if she had been, I wouldn't have tossed my aspirations by the side of the road near mile 24, as I'd done in the past. Even though it got tough to lift my waterlogged shoes and command my feet to move faster, the ultimate goal wasn't too heavy to carry the whole way.

Run LIKE THIS MOTHER
HOW TO TRAIN YOUR CHEERING SECTION

Given how noisy my kids are—can you hear them bickering from where you are sitting?—you'd think they'd be natural-born cheerleaders. But, surprisingly, they wouldn't make the cut on any pep squad.

As I learned in my two home-state marathons, Eugene in 2009 and Portland the following year, my kids are struck silent when I run by them in a race. Maybe the pressure is too great: They can barely squeak out a "Go, Mama," let alone something original or slightly inspirational. And my husband is forever stuck on, "Go, Champy!" (Champy is my sports nickname . . . long story.) I now realize I need to prep them very specifically for what I need during a race. Let my list help you, too.

SIGNS

Few things are more adorable or inspirational than a homemade sign held aloft by a tot on the side of a racecourse. Encourage your kiddies to start making them at the start of your taper. Trust me: If you leave it until the night before, the kids will be empty-handed on the sidelines; pasta preparation trumps helping with posters. Give your fans free rein with creativity, but emphasize you'll be streaking by so quickly, you won't be able to read more than a few words. Ten words max—five is better—in bold, bright colors with some eye-catching images (hearts and stick figures anyone?).

BALLOONS

When I visualize my family and friends standing by on the course sidelines, I spy them from a half-mile away, and we exchange meaningful, heartfelt comments before I even reach them. In reality, even when I know their exact geo coordinate, I frantically search the crowd for a familiar face—and often miss folks. If there are going to be a fair number of spectators, have yours hold a few balloons, a colored umbrella, or a flag so you can easily spot them. Sounds like overkill, but when you see the red heart-shaped balloons and know your fan club will soon erupt just for you, the trip to the Dollar Tree seems worth it.

PHYSICAL CONTACT

In races, Dim and I are all about high fives. Kids, grown-ups, friends, strangers: We're not picky about whose raised hand we slap. There's something about the resounding smack of flesh on flesh that gets us fired up. I'm even a fan of hugs from folks I know. That momentary reassurance and warmth is sometimes all I need to recharge my failing battery. With your family, plan in advance how much love will be exchanged—if you are intent on making your time goal, you might forgo a hug and kiss. You don't want teary eyes to trail after you if your kids and hubby feel snubbed. With friends or even random spectators, make your intentions abundantly clear: arms outstretched for a hug or a hand raised high to be smacked.

CHEERS

Ah, yes, the all-important words they yell out. If you're not picky like I am, simply encourage them to yell loudly and clearly, and to start by screaming your name or "Mommy" to grab your attention. But if you are a bit more demanding—I prefer "discerning"—let them know a few phrases or ideas that might get you fired up. In the first few miles of a longer race, a reminder of how much you've trained can help: "This is it, Mom. This is what you've been training for!" If your posse is positioned near an incline, they might want to yell, "Mommy, kill the hill!" In the final miles of a marathon, they can remind you, "You got it, Mom" or, "Pain is only temporary; pride is forever." (Obviously, this last one requires either some serious coaching or double digits in age.) And unless they are at the mile 13 marker of a half-marathon, please, please don't let them scream, "You're almost there!"

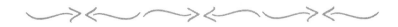

.1 RUNNING BUCKET LIST
By Dimity

We're sure another to-do list isn't on your to-do list, but in case it is, we wanted to create a bucket list that goes beyond specific races. Might we suggest you:

☐ Run a race for charity.

☐ Volunteer at a race: Manage an aid station, hand out medals, be in charge of bagels.

☐ Get a nonrunning friend to drink the Kool-Aid, then guide her through her first race. (Bonus points for letting her cross the finish line in front of you.)

☐ Plan a vacation around a race.

☐ Train for, and finish, one race that seems impossibly long to you. Might be an ultramarathon, might be a 5K.

☐ Be on a relay team, either for a marathon, triathlon, or longer 12-person relay race.

❏ Use the phrase "track workout" casually in conversation.

❏ Write down all the thoughts you have after a great run or race, then refer to them when your mojo goes MIA.

❏ Run at least a mile with one of your kids.

❏ Enter a turkey trot, a Fourth of July run, or another holiday-themed race and dress the part.

❏ Wear a shirt with your name on the front in a race so spectators can cheer for you. ("Go, Jessica!")

❏ Set a PR for new phases of your life: a decade PR, a post-pregnancy PR, a just-moved-for-the-fourth-time PR.

❏ End a run at a bar. (Drink at least one glass of water along with your other beverage of choice.)

❏ Run next to the ocean.

❏ Use a mantra in a race.

❏ Take on a trail run.

❏ Finish a race with nothing left in your tank.

❏ Run in a bigger, shorter race—in other words, have no personal space as you navigate the miles—like the Peachtree Road Race 10K (Atlanta), Bolder Boulder 10K (Colorado), Boilermaker 15K (Utica, New York), or Lilac Bloomsday Run 12K (Spokane, Washington).

❏ Drop trou (or pull aside your skirt) midrun or pre-race to pee.

❏ Run on foreign soil. (Bonus points if it's also on a different continent.)

❏ Tack on an extra mile or two to your run just because you feel like it.

❏ Know all the words to your favorite psych-up song so well, you can sing it to yourself when a battery dies.

❏ Run at night, guided either by a full moon or a headlamp.

❏ Come home from a winter run with sweat icicles on your hat (or, better yet, your eyelashes).

❏ Get injured—then stage a comeback.

❏ Register for a race the day before, just because you feel like it.

And space for a few entries of your own.

_____

_____

_____

_____

13

RACE DAY: **THE FINAL COUNTDOWN**

By Dimity + Sarah

The work is done; the cows are in the barn; it's taper time, gals. Because you know nearly every running-related detail of our lives, we thought we'd share with you the prep work and thoughts we have leading up to a half-marathon, which we're pretending starts at 7 A.M. on a Sunday. (Visualize along with us: We're also imagining we each take first in our age groups and knock substantial times off our respective PRs, thanks to our amazing training and preparation.)

T MINUS 7 DAYS

Dimity: Head over to weather.com and start to check the forecast obsessively, or at least four times a day up until race day. Each time, I'm slightly bummed there isn't an hourly weather map available yet for Sunday's race.

T MINUS 5 DAYS

Dimity: Get slightly concerned my training isn't going to kick in. I know taper time, when miles are minimal, is when my mind goes even more into overdrive, so I try to take that into account, but my legs don't feel as fresh as I think they should by now. They always come around by race day, but I wish there was some gas gauge–like window on my quads to allow me to see them getting revved.

SBS: Shooting out some e-mails to rustle up a playdate for race-day afternoon for at least one of the kiddos, thus ensuring less chaos in the house. Maybe I'll even be able to slip in a nap. (The mere thought makes me redouble my e-mail efforts.)

Despite being on deadline for a *Runner's World* article, I spend at least 20 minutes studying the racecourse. Like my older daughter, Phoebe, prepping for her weekly spelling test, I want to make sure I know things backward and forward. Does that long hill start at mile 8, or end there? At what street is the turnaround before we head back toward the finish line?

T MINUS 4 DAYS

Dimity: After checking the weather for the third time today, I head to my drawer o' spandex and see what outfit I want to wear. Unlike a certain someone—ahem, SBS—I don't have specific race outfits, although these days I run in some kind of shirt from the Another Mother Runner collection. When I'm dragging, and somebody yells, "You're one badass mother runner!" or laughs at my shirt, I get a momentary boost.

To make sure I'm covered, I will wash all of my favorite sports bras, as well as two bottoms (one pair of capris, one skirt).

SBS: Laundry day here in Portland, where it takes workout clothes a good two days to air dry. Wash several skirts as I debate patterned versus dependable black. Give a whiff to my wool arm warmers: slightly pungent, but not overly ripe. Leave them out, but toss in several bras, as I want to wear one that makes me look slightly bodacious under my AMR tank.

T MINUS 3 DAYS

SBS: Blow off boot camp. If Ashleigh has us do too many lunges and squats, my legs will be toast. Right about now is when I start consciously conserving my energy and being kind to my legs. When I hear the UPS guy knock on the front door, I forgo answering it. I know he'll leave the package without a signature, resulting in one fewer set of stairs I have to tromp up and down.

When I'm in the kitchen at lunchtime, eating leftover pizza, I check the cupboards to make sure I have all the ingredients for my race-morning smoothie, plus good bread for toast. I add bananas to my grocery list, as I want to ensure they are the perfect ripeness on Sunday morning.

T MINUS 2 DAYS

SBS: It's gadget time. I spend way too much time making the. perfect. playlist. Maybe it's a little heavy on the Fitz & The Tantrums songs, but they put a spring in my step. Then I connect the iPod to download my "Half-Marathon Heaven" playlist and charge the device, which reminds me to plug in my Garmin. Got to be sure all batteries—not just my body's—are fully charged.

T MINUS 36 HOURS

SBS: Knowing it's the sleep you get *two* nights pre-race, not the night of, that can make or break

TAKE IT *From* A MOTHER
HOW WOULD YOU DESCRIBE YOUR RACING STYLE?

"Slow and steady. I like to get my money's worth from every course!"

—KRISTINE (Strangest thing seen on a run: It's a tie between two deer having a *National Geographic* moment and a man running naked.)

"I'm a bit of a rabbit, unfortunately, because I just feel so good after a nice taper. This has never proved truly disastrous for me, but I'm sure my times would be faster if I could learn to control it!"

—PHOEBE (Loved running alongside a friend for the pal's first race, because "I was able to mix the encouraging friend part of me with my 'Get 'er done, dammit' coach part.")

"Run fast and don't fall down."

—SUZANNE (Took this advice from her now 7-year-old daughter, who was 3 at the time.)

"Slow."

—STEPHANIE ("I think I like saying 'I'm a runner' more than I like running. I hope that's not weird.")

"Competitive, but I know my limits."

—BOBBI (Takes out her earbuds during races if somebody strikes up a conversation.)

"Enjoy every mile."

—HENRIETTAE (Loves hearing the national anthem before a race starts.)

"I am competitive, but only with myself. I love to encourage other runners who seem defeated."

—TRACY (Race-day philosophy: If you're physically prepared, it's 90 percent mind over matter.)

"Laid-back but persistent."

—AMY (Doesn't run through injury: "At first twinge, I'm taking a break.")

"Fly and die. I am not one of those people who can sprint the last quarter-mile of a race."

—RACHEL (Was once chased by a pack of Chihuahuas while on vacation. "It was the fastest mile I ever ran.")

"Neo-conservative borderline trashy? I don't think I know what a racing style is."

—AMANDA (Entertains herself on long runs by taking photos with her iPhone and using Facebook. "Seriously.")

race-day performance, I get a bit anxious around 8:45. I decide tonight's the night to pop an Ambien to ensure sweet slumber. Ear plugs and "Hollywood shades" complete my sleep kit.

Dimity: As I wait for my Tylenol PM to kick in, I settle on two potential outfits. Capris, tank, and long-sleeve tech tee if it's below 50—I'll tie the tee around my waist if I get hot—and skirt, tank, and long sleeve if it's between 50 and 60.

T MINUS 24 HOURS

SBS: After a short, easy, shake-out-the-legs run, I shave my 'pits and legs. Wishing I'd remembered to apply it sooner, I slather on some self-tanner. Wonder if there's enough time to give a glow to my pale gams?

Speaking of color, I've been paying careful attention to the shade of my urine. What hue *is* pale straw, anyway? I decide pee the color of Crystal Light Lemonade is fine for letting me know I'm well hydrated.

Dimity: Head to the expo to pick up my number. As I walk around the expo, I peruse the schwag bag slyly so that it doesn't look like I only race for mini Luna Bars and free GU, which, truth be told, I kind of do. I head to the T-shirt table and check out the tees. If they're unisex or ugly, I usually opt not to take one, or, if possible, I'll grab a smaller size so one of my kids can use it for PJs. I've taken too many shirts I didn't like on sight, then had them clutter up my dresser before donating them to Goodwill. If I'm with a friend, we may peruse the booths, but I'm usually an in-and-out kind of girl. I'd rather shop for running clothes and shoes when I don't have a race hanging over my head.

SBS: I take the kids to the playground, resisting the strong urge to take a nap. (I don't want to mess with my ability to fall asleep tonight—no sleep aids for me the night before a race.) I plant myself on a shady bench and read the *New York Times* on my phone, refusing to push my kids on the tire swing for fear I'll wrench my back. For Mama, this visit is all about resting, not playing.

T MINUS 12 HOURS

Dimity: Definitely have one beer and plenty of water with my dinner, usually pasta with veggies and a salad. Then indulge in dessert, ideally a piece of carrot cake. Never know what may happen tomorrow, so I might as well enjoy tonight.

T MINUS 10 HOURS

Dimity: After checking the hourly forecast for the last time tonight, I solidify my outfit choice. I lay the tank flat on my bed and position my race number squarely in the middle of the bottom half.

Without letting the bib shift a centimeter, I fasten all four pins, then pick up the tank. The number, without fail, is slanted or off center. C'est la vie.

T MINUS 9 HOURS, 30 MINUTES

Dimity: Climb into bed at 9:30, my usual bedtime, and pretend like I don't have a race tomorrow. Good luck with that, says my mind.

T MINUS 5 HOURS

Dimity: After tossing and turning and finally falling asleep around midnight, I wake up about 2 A.M. feeling like my bladder might explode. Empty it and think, *only 3½ hours of sleep left. Get back to sleep, ASAP!*

T MINUS 2.5 HOURS

Dimity: Rise and shine. Or snooze a few times, then rise and shine. I first head downstairs to get breakfast and some water boiling for tea: want to rouse the intestines so that I can use my home bathroom. Check the weather again, and promise myself it's the final time.

PRACTICAL *Motherly* ADVICE
RACE-DAY CHECK LIST

ITEM	SBS SAYS . . .	DIMITY SAYS . . .
Race number	Pinned to skirt or capris so I can mop sweaty face with tee.	Always goes on top, not bottom, where it bugs me.
Shoes	Used to race (and do speedwork) in flexible, lightweight beauts . . . until they contributed to my plantar fasciitis.	I race in what I train in. No special kicks for me.
Socks	Drymax Maximum Protection Running Socks: guaranteed blister guards.	Balegas are my fave. Worth the extra $$.
Bottom of some sort	Donated all my shorts years ago. Skirts are my three-season friends; capris only when it's 50 degrees or colder. Never tights. (I've got hot legs.)	Skirt = summertime. Capris = leaves are falling. Tights = snow is blowing. Tights and capris must be black to hide any bodily fluids that might escape.
Undies	One word: commando.	One word: ditto.
Sports bra	Prefer back clasp to avoid sweaty overhead-shimmy post-race.	Gotta have padding; hate the headlights.

ITEM	SBS SAYS . . .	DIMITY SAYS . . .
Top of some sort	Coordinated with my skirt or capris: I'm a fastinista.	Tank: summer Long-sleeve tee: fall/winter/spring.
Hat or visor	Visors don't look cute on this short-haired lass.	Ditto. I rock a hat in summer, or my face is awash in sweat.
Gloves	Critical even in moderate temps as I suffer from Raynaud's disease (my fingers hurt and turn white).	Thin ones for winter races; tuck them in tights' waistband when I get warm.
Arm warmers	Swear by them, both for warmth and style points.	Never worn 'em in a race. I feel like I need to be faster to do so.
Sunglasses	It has to be blindingly bright for me to race in them, but I always sport a brimmed hat.	Hat is enough in the summer, bandana and shades for other three seasons.
Music	Can't. Live. Without.	The bigger the race, the less I can handle tunes. Too much stimulation.
Garmin or watch	A Garmin, but only look at it 1/100th as often as Dimity does during a race.	Sometimes, but I do get obsessive. I also like to run with my wrists naked.
Hydration belt	It's not a good look for me (belly bulge), but I like carrying my own fluids, gels, and nano in an Amphipod.	Nope.
Calories for the race	I'm religious about fueling—with GU or Roctane—at specific points (like mile 4, 8, and 11 of a half).	Stash a gel—my fave is Espresso Love or Chocolate GU—or two in my skirt pocket.
Extra layer of clothing	Can't stand to be hot. Would rather be shivering at the start than dripping by mile 2. If it's too chilly, I wear a tossable tee.	Usually wear a warm layer on top to the race, then check it.
Change of clothing, post-race	Gotta get out of sweaty bra posthaste to prevent excessive chills.	If I remember and I have a car; not for away races.
Directions to race	Reason #7,874 why I love my iPhone.	Let's just say I like to stress myself out, pre-race. I consider multiple U-turns, which cause me to sweat, my warm-up.
Knowledge of racecourse	Studying course and elevation map: favorite workday time waster in weeks pre-race.	Ignorance is bliss. Until that hellish hill at mile 4.
Jacket or vest	I swear by vests in my training life, but never race in any outerwear.	Not a vest girl. Usually a light jacket in winter; I like two layers for colder races.
Phone	Once it directs me to the race, it stays stashed in the car.	Never run with it; usually leave it in the car.
Cash or credit card	I travel light: no to both.	Never run with it; usually leave it in the car.
Car or hotel key	In Amphipod belt.	Don't stash hotel key in your sports bra. Serious chafe.
Sunscreen	No: As an Oregonian, I have to soak up vitamin D whenever I can.	Always on my face (below my eyes), sometimes on arms and legs depending on the season.
BodyGlide	Nearly as critical as race chip. Upper thighs, rib cage under bra strap, underside of upper arms. Chafing is the devil.	Hardly ever use it during a race; sometimes regret forgetting it.

SBS: Wake up a few minutes before alarm sounds, hop out of bed to brush my teeth, and peer out bedroom window to determine weather. As usual, the mere act of standing in the morning gets things moving. Poop for first of what ends up being three times this morning.

Strip off pajamas to begin the anti-chafing ritual. It begins, easily enough, with swipes of Body-Glide. Then comes the layered effect with broad swaths of Asics Chafe Free; applying the chalky white liquid is like whitewashing my inner thighs. Yes, the process takes almost as long as the actual race, but this combo is my no-fail, anti-chafe strategy.

T MINUS 30 MINUTES

Dimity: I arrive at the racecourse about 30 minutes before the gun goes off. I like to have enough time to drop a bag, get in line for the Porta-Potty, and soak in a little of the atmosphere, but I don't like to be there with too much time to spare, or I'll get too nervous or cold.

First, I drop my bag. Although I like to travel lightly, after a fall race I know I'll want my fleece jacket. If you're racing with a bunch of people, consolidate your items into one or two bags, then have the fastest runner check it. She can grab it and have your goodies waiting for you at the finish line.

Then I scope out the Porta-Potty line. If it looks ridiculously long, I'll investigate other options. If I'm only going number 1, I check to see if there are any woods or out-of-the-way fields around. If not, I'll bide my time and hope the line moves as urgently as I have to pee.

SBS: I walk a block or two away from the race hoopla before starting my warm-up of easy running, then strides. I try not to attract attention to myself, as I don't resemble the slight, fleet-feeted runners who bust out aggressive warm-ups. I'm just looking to work out a few kinks and break a light sweat.

Afterward, I pick up my Amphipod belt and make sure a Roctane is in the outside mesh pocket for easy access at mile 4. With 10 minutes left to the start, I pop two pieces of Jolt Energy Gum into my mouth. Caffeine is my now-not-so-secret race-day boost since I otherwise eschew it.

T MINUS 7 OR SO MINUTES

Dimity: Jump in the corral and make sure my two GUs aren't hanging out of my pocket. If I'm alone, I may strike up a conversation with a fellow runner, or I may hang solo. Depends on how I feel. I definitely like to line up toward one edge of the road, leaving me more personal space.

SBS: I "pardon me, excuse me" my way to the middle of the appropriate starting corral. Once situated, I stand stock still with my elbow cocked, locking in a satellite signal on my GPS. Then I shift my attention to my nano, checking for the, oh, 78th time it's *not* set on shuffle so that Fitz and his fellows will come on at the precise moment I planned midrace. I thread my Yurbuds cord under my bra strap and down my shirt, then plug it into my iPod. I cue up "Half-Marathon Heaven," and I'm ready to go.

Dimity: I'm as ready as I'll ever be. Let's get this party started.

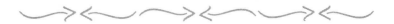

.1 WHEN I CROSS A FINISH LINE I FEEL . . .

"Unstoppable." —Marci

"Relief." —Karen

"Like I can conquer the world and anything it throws at me." —Rachel

"An immediate urge to hit the restroom for some sour tummy relief." —Emily

"Great, but wondering if I left some in the tank." —Christy

"Like I'm going to die." —Jane

"Victorious, even though I haven't won." —Lesley

"Thankful, exhausted, and ready for a beer." —Lauren

"Like I might cry." —Tyler

"Strong and alive." —Carolina

"Emotionally full." —Kelly

"Invincible." —Bobby

"Happy and grateful" —Robin

"Like a champion! Like a badass mother runner! Oh, and sorta like I want to drop . . . but that's normal, right?!" —Kelly

"Thankful I can run." —Amanda

"In disbelief I did it." —Nina

"Exuberant! Exhilarated! Energized!" —Carol

"Like I have accomplished something for myself." —Rene

"Honestly, a little queasy. A sense of satisfaction usually takes a few hours to settle into my bones." —Kate

"Very emotional." —Tracey

"Like a superstar!" —Amber

"Happy to be done and happy to have done it." —Molly

"Competent." —Terri

"Complete." —Kendra

"High." —Angie

"Untouchable. Free. Fast." —Maria

"Like I can do anything. Except run any farther." —Stephanie

"Overflowing with happiness, exhaustion, pride, relief, you name it." —Lesley

"Insanely proud." —Nicole

"So glad it's over! And within 30 minutes, ready to train for the next race." —Katrina

"What all of you said." —Dimity + Sarah

ACKNOWLEDGMENTS

From Dimity

I am, as always, indebted to and in love with my husband, Grant. He pumps me up when I need it, gracefully knocks me down—not literally—when I need it, and gets the kids breakfast six out of seven days of the week so I can get my sweat on. I'm still not sure sometimes why he puts up with me, but I'm so grateful he does.

Ms. Poppers and Mr. Pie, you are in my heart and in every step.

Thank you Mom and John for your office space, your open fridge and tab, and the support and love you continue to pour on my family and me. We are so lucky.

Megan and Sarah: Love you both to pieces, but please know that I'm still holding out for a 40th birthday half-marathon. When you read this, the day will be just 2 months away, so start planning—and training—if you haven't. Jeff and Tom: Thank you in advance for letting them go.

I love my ladies with whom I trot around the neighborhood: Laurel, LeAnn, Becky, Katherine, Bine, Kelly, Lisa, Jenni—and the four-legged man of the group, Copper. Thanks for laughing and lunging with me. I also heart running with Erin, Sarah, Amanda, and the Stroller Strides crowd, especially because I don't have to push one anymore. Thanks to Katie and Pip, whose presence in my life has deepened my perspective for the places running can take you. And gratitude to Briana, who has patience in spades and has almost made me love fast pickups.

SBS, my sister from another mother: May we have many more words, miles, shopping trips to Anthropologie, and chuckles together.

From **Sarah**

Loving thanks to my husband, who I believe was inspired by *Run Like a Mother* to become a devoted gym goer. Jack, our feelings toward a treadmill might differ, but our shared sense of humor unites us.

Phoebe, John, and Daphne: I love you with all my heart to infinity.

I couldn't have written this book without the support of my parents, especially their taking care of three little folk while I was holed up at various Connecticut libraries.

Courtenay: *RLAM*-related travel (and our sets of twins) reunited us, and I love you now even more than I did in high school, if that's possible.

I've become a more social runner, in large part thanks to my friends from carpooling, Molly and Heidi. I'll see you on my corner at 6 A.M. And, Sheila, it was such fun traveling the road to the 2010 Portland Marathon with you.

I am filled with gratitude for countless reasons when I think of Joanne Godfrey, but the stand-out one is for being the most ebullient cheerleader a BQ-aspirant could ever hope to have at my three, count 'em, most recent marathons. (Third time was the charm, Jo!)

I'm thankful for the Internet—and the AMR community—for giving me Phoebe, Alison, and Ginny, who brighten my semi-hermetic days with e-mails.

To Megan, Ashley, Julie, Meredith, Eryn, and the rest of the Vancouver posse: You make me feel funny, fast, younger, and, above all, cherished. I feel blessed to be part of your world.

Most of all, I am grateful for my sister from another mother runner, Dimity. The fact we were still laughing on Labor Day sums up, for me, why we work so well together.

From Dimity and Sarah

We've got to start by saying a ginormous thanks—which doesn't feel like it's big enough—to the amazing tribe of women who have created the Another Mother Runner community and the supportive, funny, honest vibe that lives there. (Dang it that we can't sometimes actually *live* there.) Although we'd happily log a few miles with any of you, we're particularly indebted to the more than 300 of you who took precious time out of your days to fill out a ridiculously long survey that provided the fodder for the "Take It from a Mother" (TIFAM) columns and the occasional, but very necessary, inspiration for us to keep writing. We wish we could've put about 35 more TIFAM columns in this book, but then it would be the size of a dictionary and couldn't be wedged into your purse to read at soccer practice.

To Jane Dystel, our agent, we are grateful for your continued support; to our editor, Chris Schillig, your confidence in our ideas and abilities allows us to be a great team. This book wouldn't have had life breathed into it if not for the devoted support of our publicist, Kathy Hilliard, and Amy Worley, Andrews McMeel's social-media maven.

Many, many thanks to our "genius" intern, Jessie, for your enthusiastic, self-starter work and technical support. (And Sarah loves laughing and chatting with you in her kitchen.)

We'd love to give running coach Christine Hinton a hug in person (one day!). She wrote all the innovative, efficient training plans in this book, turned them in way before her deadline, then was beyond patient, when, 3 months later, we barraged her with questions and edits and pleas to look over our renditions of them.

To the other experts who contributed so helpfully and generously—Ivana Bisaro, Jeff Galloway, Janet Hamilton, Sarah Johnson, Ilana Katz, Ashleigh Kayser, and Sage Rountree—thank you for your time and expertise.

Finally, a shout-out to Katie Oglesby, Amanda Upson, and Cathy Zielske, who, in their individual ways, contributed more to this book and the AMR community than they realize. We are so appreciative for your insights and wit.

RUNNING RESOURCES

A helpful, but by no means exhaustive, list of resources we've found valuable both professionally and personally.

PEOPLE

Ivana Bisaro, a member of the army of coaches at Carmichael Training Systems, can whip you into marathon shape even if you have a stress fracture. Find her at www.trainright.com.

Jeff Galloway, an Olympian and pioneer in the running world, has training plans, retreats, and camps, plus books galore. Find him at www.jeffgalloway.com.

Janet Hamilton, a running coach and exercise physiologist, has an encyclopedic knowledge about how the running human body works. She's at www.runningstrong.com.

Christine Hinton, a running coach and ultrarunner, crafted all the training plans in this book. In a word, she rocks—and can get you to, too. Find her at www.therunningcoach.com and at www.thepregnantrunner.com.

Ilana Katz, a nutritionist and Ironman, could talk about carbs, protein, and fat—and how to use them to help your running—in her sleep. Check her out at www.onforlife.com.

Sage Rountree, a renowned yogini, triathlete, runner, and coach, can power up your quads, release your hamstrings, and make you smile along the way. She's at www.sagerountree.com.

HOW-TO RUNNING BOOKS

The Athlete's Guide to Recovery: Rest, Relax & Restore for Peak Performance, by Sage Rountree. Boulder, Colo.: Velo Press, 2011.

Barefoot Running Step by Step: Barefoot Ken Bob, the Guru of Shoeless Running, Shares His Personal Technique for Running with More Speed, Less Impact, Fewer Injuries, and More Fun, by Ken Bob Saxton and Roy M. Wallack. Beverly, Mass.: Fair Winds Press, 2011.

ChiRunning: A Revolutionary Approach to Effortless, Injury-Free Running, by Danny Dreyer and Katherine Dreyer. New York: Simon & Schuster, 2009.

Nancy Clark's Sports Nutrition Guidebook, by Nancy Clark. Champaign, Ill.: Human Kinetics, 2008.

Natural Running: The Simple Path to Stronger, Healthier Running, by Danny Abshire and Brian Metzler. Boulder, Colo.: Velo Press, 2010.

Run: The Mind–Body Method of Running by Feel, by Matt Fitzgerald. Boulder, Colo.: Velo Press, 2010.

Running Doc's Guide to Healthy Running: How to Fix Injuries, Stay Active, and Run Pain-Free, by Lewis G. Maharam, MD. Boulder, Colo.: Velo Press, 2011.

INSPIRING SPORTS BOOKS

The Amateurs: The Story of Four Young Men and Their Quest for an Olympic Gold Medal, by David Halberstam. New York: Ballantine Books, 1996. Pulitzer Prize winner David Halberstam breathes exquisite life into this account of a quartet of male rowers striving to make the 1984 Olympics team. (This book was Sarah's bible when she was a rower at Colgate.)

Born to Run: A Hidden Tribe, Superathletes, and the Greatest Race the World Has Never Seen, by Christopher McDougall. New York: Knopf, 2009. A book that incited a barefoot revolution. While we might not buy everything McDougall recommends—neither of us will ever run sans shoes—it's a fun read.

Let's Take the Long Way Home: A Memoir of Friendship. by Gail Caldwell. New York: Random House, 2011. Not a triumphant sports tale, but rather one about two women who bond over their love of rowing, dogs, writing, and past addictions. A testament to the strength of female friendship.

Marathon Woman: Running the Race to Revolutionize Women's Sports, by Kathrine Switzer. Cambridge, Mass.: Da Capo Press, 2009. The well-told story of Switzer, who, wearing a hooded sweatshirt and sweatpants, broke male-only barriers in the Boston Marathon, and continued running strong. Whether you know it or not, Switzer is likely the reason you're racing today.

Mile Markers: The 26.2 Most Important Reasons Why Women Run, by Kristin Armstrong. Emmaus, Penn.: Rodale, 2011. Tales from a woman whose thoughts run as quickly as her feet—and regularly echo through our heads.

Open: An Autobiography, by Andre Agassi. New York: Vintage, 2010. A surprisingly great book that delves into everything from Andre's hatred of tennis and his domineering father to his marriage to Steffi Graf.

Personal Record: A Love Affair with Running, by Rachel Toor. Lincoln, Neb.: University of Nebraska Press, 2008. Twenty-six chapters about running, relationships, and life by a talented writer. (And .2 to finish things off.)

Swimming to Antarctica: Tales of a Long-Distance Swimmer, by Lynne Cox. Orlando, Fla.: Harcourt, 2005. A very talented writer—the *New Yorker* published her articles about her adventures—Cox swims in places most people wouldn't dare to dip a toe.

What I Talk About When I Talk About Running: A Memoir, by Haruki Murakami. Translated by Philip Gabriel. New York: Knopf, 2008. Murakami, an acclaimed Japanese writer, started running at age 33. This insightful read makes us glad he laced up.

ANOTHER MOTHER RUNNER DICTIONARY[1]

10 percent rule: An oft-cited injury-prevention tenet stating you shouldn't increase your weekly mileage or intensity by more than 10 percent. So if you're currently running 20 miles, don't bump up to any more than 22 miles next week. Or if you've run 20 miles this week, but haven't done any speedwork or tempo runs, do no more than 2 miles next week at a pumped-up pace—and keep your total mileage at 20.

400: Once around a regulation track, measured in meters.

800: Twice around a regulation track, measured in meters.

1,000: Two and a half times around a regulation track, measured in meters.

1,200: Three times around a regulation track, measured in meters.

1,600: One mile, or four times, on a regulation track. Measured in—say it with us—meters. (It's a little short of 1 mile, but we're not arguing with the standard.)

A

AMR: Another mother runner.

Athena: A supposedly flattering term for larger female athletes, usually those who weigh more than 150 pounds. Bigger races—and many triathlons—have an Athena (or "Filly") division, so us heavier gals don't have to compete against the wisps whose legs are roughly the circumference of our forearms. The male version of the Athena is a Clydesdale, which makes Athena seem not so bad, right?

---

[1] A mix of serious running terms, which you can drop into conversations without hesitation ("Oh, my 6 x 800 session at the track really gave me a massive lactic acid burn, but I felt so good, I even finished with some strides."), and many more entertaining terms from the AMR tribe, which we compiled via a blog post long ago.

B

BAMR: Badass mother runner.

Bandit: An unregistered runner in a race who didn't pay the entry fee. We know it's tempting, but we can't condone being one of these bad guys.

Barnacle buster: Any thing/person/activity used to distract, deter, and detach one's children from one's legs, thus freeing a mother for a run.

BBTN: Barely better than nothing—a description of just-got-out-there run.

Bonk: A condition marked by a massive decrease in pace, motivation, and control over one's legs and caused by depletion of energy, or glycogen, stores in the muscles. Usually occurs around mile 20 of a marathon, but can pop up in most any race or long run. Consuming calories, such as a gel or a sports drink, can help you bounce back somewhat, but you'll still suffer for the remainder of your miles. Avoid bonking by racing a smart race—see **even split** or **negative split**—and eating along the way. *Synonym:* hitting the wall.

BQ: What some runners pursue as fervently as 10-year-olds beg to get a cell phone. It's a speedy marathon time that qualifies a runner to gain entry to the famed Boston Marathon. Times are based on age and gender. For example, a woman aged 35 to 39 needs to run 3:40:00 or faster to BQ.

BRF: Best running friend.

Bublé effect: When a song sneaks its way into your iPod and puts you to sleep/mellows out your run faster than a Michael Bublé song.

C

Cadence: The number of times your feet strike the ground during 1 minute of running. Most running experts recommend aiming for about 180 steps per minute—or having each foot hit the ground 90 times. (If you're over 5 feet 10 inches, you can lower your count to about 174.) To figure out your cadence, you can geek out like Dimity does and use a metronome, or you can count the number of times your right foot hits the ground in 20 seconds and multiply by 3. Most people have too low of a cadence; to increase yours, think about shortening your stride to an almost alarming degree.

Caffeine jolt: Temporary acceleration produced when you see a runner—usually a cute, younger, faster man—you want to impress.

Carbo-load: The best part of marathon training. During the final few days of your taper, when your miles are minimal, you up the carbohydrates—rice, pasta, bread, simple fruits and veggies like bananas and corn—in your diet to as much as 90 percent of what you consume. Doing so fills up and tops out the glycogen (or fuel) stores in your muscles, so that your quads' needle is on "F" when you hit the starting line.

Character builders: Hill workouts, any speedwork over 400 meters, or runs in extreme heat/cold.

Chip timed: What all but the most homegrown of races are these days. With an electronic sensor (aka a "chip") affixed to your ankle, shoelaces, or the back of your race bib, your race time is automagically recorded. (And sometimes even transmitted to the race website in real-time stats, as happens in some bigger marathons.) The chip eliminates the need when you cross the finish line to immediately press the stop button on your Garmin or watch, which, it should be noted, ruins your finisher's photo.

Chunk change: The extra poundage you carry around in your own personal trunk.

Church: Virtual place/real route many **BAMR'ers** go on Sunday morning, the only time they can fit in a long run.

Coin slot: Body part that shows when low-cut running shorts are too overloaded with GU, keys, and music player.

Cooldown: The thing you're so sorely tempted to skip at the end of a workout, especially after a tough one like a tempo run or track session. Resist the urge: It helps your heart rate and breathing return closer to normal, and clears the (painful) lactic acid out of your legs.

Creepers: Shorts that don't stay in place.

Crop dusting: Passing gas on the run.

Crotch rot: Dripping-wet running tights.

Cutdown: A run during which you progressively get faster—or cut down—your pace. Depending on the length of the run, the miles could be faster by as little as 10 seconds or as much as 45 seconds. Helps with learning pacing, as in, "Oh, this is what a 9:30-minute mile feels like."

Cycling Casanovas: Guys biking on the trails with waaaaaay too much cologne on. (Or who are waaaaaay too into themselves and their overlogoed jerseys.)

D

Dehydration station: Water stop.

DFL: Dead, um, *Freakin'* Last. You may be last in a race, as a runner, but you're a winner in the race of life. Cheesy, but very true.

Dip dye: Phenomenon that occurs when your sweat-soaked shirt starts to visibly dampen your shorts/tights/skirt from the waist, slowly working its way down.

DNF: Did Not Finish. Yes, it's not the greatest thing to see next to your name in the race results, but consider the alternative: DNS. As in Did Not Start.

Dory run: Tough run, where just getting through it is a victory. Stems from the movie *Finding Nemo*, in which Dory says, "Just keep swimming. Just keep swimming."

Double flush: Sign of an effective colon evacuation.

Dreadmill: Affectionate term for the treadmill.

Dropping the kids off at the pool: Pre-run evac in the bathroom. Might be followed by a **double flush**.

Dynamic stretching: Stretches that involve swinging your arms and legs in a controlled manner to gently increase your range of motion and get your juices flowing. Usually done pre-run for a simple warm-up.

E

Empty the tank: To cross the finish line having expended all energy your body has to offer. It's the aim of SBS in almost every race, and something Dimity isn't really interested in doing in this lifetime.

Endorphins: Feel-good amino acids, produced when you exercise, that are responsible for the elusive "runner's high."

Entourage: Young passengers in a single, double, or—you're our hero—triple running stroller. *Synonym:* portable cheering section.

Even split: Running at a pace so that each mile, give or take a few seconds, takes about as long as the previous one. A good race strategy for a beginner or somebody taking on a distance for the first time.

F

Fancy pants: Capris or tights with reflective stripes. (Or any favorite bottoms you reserve for race day.)

Fartlek: Smirk-inducing Swedish word meaning a short burst of speed that gets thrown into a random run for "fun." You can fartlek from one telephone pole to another, or up to a tree in the distance, or past a park bench. Then you ease back on the pace, and, given that it was such a riot, do it a couple more times. Because SBS encourages her kids to say "pass gas" instead of *that* "f" word—or, worse, "toot"— we generally opted to call them "intervals" in this book.

Finishing kick: The last part of a race, when you turn up your pace as much as possible until you cross the finish line. When you start your kick is up to you: Dimity prefers to kick it in with less than .2 mile to go of any race; SBS tries to do it for at least the last half mile, if not a little more.

FIRM: Friends in Running + Motherhood. (See also **AMR.**)

Full moon rising: condition when shorts or skirt head south during a run.

G

Galloway: An outing during which you run and walk at specific increments, like run for 6 minutes, walk for 1, repeat until run is done. Named after Jeff Galloway, father of the run/walk method.

Glucose: What glycogen is called when it's stored in the bloodstream; the amount in the blood is fairly low, compared with your muscle stores.

Glycogen: The fuel, stored in your muscles and liver and created by converting carbs, that your body uses to run.

Go Fasters: Running shoes.

Googly eyes: When nipples, which are a little past their prime, aren't "looking forward" anymore.

GU-doo: Product of intestinal distress brought about by consuming GU. Or the act of depositing the product of intestinal distress in a Porta-Potty.

H

Heel damage: Calluses that never clear up.

HFH: Holy Frackin' Hill. How runners/tweeters, especially in western Pennsylvania, describe their runs. (Example: I did 5 #HFHs on lunchtime run. #legsaretoast)

Hill repeats: Repetitions of, um, hills. Seriously, though, these are a highly effective way to build leg strength and speed without hitting the track. Involves tackling numerous (four to 10-plus) hills of various degrees of steepness. Charge up; trot back down; charge up; trot back down . . . you get the picture.

Hitting the wall: See **bonk**.

HR: Heart rate. It's what gets elevated when you run (or think about Ryan Reynolds). Often used as HRM, for heart rate monitor.

Hungry butt: When underwear rides up your crack while running.

Hungry thighs: When your shorts bulge up between your legs.

I

Involuntary speedwork: Increased pace brought on by significant other pacing in the driveway, needing to leave for work.

J

Jet propelled: Description for a gaseous run. (Unfortunately, does not typically make the runner faster.)

Jogging: A term we aren't even going to define—and you are not allowed to use. If you propel yourself forward faster than a walk, you are *running*.

Jog itch: Condition that occurs after having a good run; all of a sudden, you can't wait for your next. Also, the feeling you get when you're injured and can't run. Or you're housebound with three kids under 7 and can't run. Or you're stuck in a meeting and can't run. Or . . .

Junk holders: Liners on men's running shorts.

K

K: Kilometer, which is the equivalent of .62 mile. (Yes, the world should be on one system.)

L

Lactic acid: A chemical substance that forms in your muscles when you run at a pace that you can't breathe easily, and you definitely can't talk. Makes your legs feel like they are burning.

Ladder: A track workout in which the distances go up, and then down, like (hottie) firefighters on a ladder. A typical ladder might be 1 minute, 2 minutes, 3 minutes, 2 minutes, 1 minute; with recovery between each effort. While they seem complicated on paper, ladders are more interesting to do than, say, 10 x 1 minute, and once you're on the way back "down," life feels pretty good. The key with running ladder intervals is adjusting your effort, or pace, as the distance changes. The shorter the interval, the harder the effort. Longer segments should be approached in a more controlled manner.

Land mines: Dog poop or horse manure left in the middle of a trail.

Log: What you record your runs in, whether on paper or electronically. Also what you try to avoid tripping over while trail running.

LPPM: Last Possible Pee Moment. Occurs right before you head out the door.

LSD: No, not the psychedelic drug favored by Timothy Leary and Jerry Garcia, but Long, Slow Distance, the pace the majority of your long runs should be.

M

Masters runner: A runner over the age of 40, which SBS keeps reminding herself is supposedly "the new 30." This age distinction comes into play in races (and track meets), as bigger ones have Masters divisions to keep the youngsters from taking home all the hardware.

Mountain Dew: Sweat between the boobs.

N

Naked run: A workout done with no music, no GPS, no set route.

Natural energy production: Watts produced by thighs rubbing together.

Negative split: The holy grail of racers. This elusive goal is achieved by running the second half of a race (or workout) faster than the first half, which involves pacing yourself exceptionally well and not going out too fast. We're both pretty sure it's a phenomenon we've only *read* about. (Do as we say, not as we do.)

Noassatall: Condition the rears of runners get from too many miles. *Antonym*: a J-Lo.

Nursing mom: Style achieved by a very wet sports bra and a dry shirt—and having the two meet. Two big, very pronounced circles, like your baby hasn't eaten in days.

O

OMD: Orchestral maneuvers in the dark; a run before sunrise or after sunset.

P

Pacer: A runner charged with the task of running a race in a specific amount of time, such as a 4:15 marathon or 2:00 half, to help other racers reach that goal.

Pickups: "Hey, baby, come here often?" Oh, sorry, that's a *pickup line*. Pickups are very short sprints (shorter than **fartleks**) thrown into a run that's otherwise done at an easy pace. Like a come-on from a handsome stranger in a bar, they can be a nice diversion in an otherwise ho-hum night out/run.

Prairie dogging: An urgent need to poop on a run; the matter almost escapes and then doesn't, the way a prairie dog goes in and out of his house. *Synonym*: turtle head.

PR/PB: No, not "public relations" and "peanut butter." PR = personal record, your fastest finishing time for a *recent* race. (No official statute of limitations, but don't go bragging about some sub-20:00 5K if, say, a Bush was president when you ran it.) PB = personal best, favored by our neighbors to the north in Canada.

Predator: Another runner who sneaks up on you and passes you. (After the predator passes you, you're *roadkill*.)

Priming the pistons: Applying BodyGlide to the inner thighs, the area most prone to chafing.

Puke pace: Self-explanatory. The goal during most speed workouts.

R

Race pace: The pace at which you travel between the starting line and finish line. Often a subject that requires quite a bit of discussion and obsessive thought. To determine yours, check out the Magic Mile on page 106.

Rart: Running fart.

Recovery run: A short, easy cruise, usually under 3 miles, you do the day after a hard effort or race. Meant to get healing blood flowing to your aching muscles. (You'll feel much better afterward, we promise.)

Repeats: A way to describe a workout in which you run the same preset distance more than once. Although you can do 400 or 800 repeats, the term is usually applied to the mile distance (for example, "mile repeats" and the dreaded "2-mile repeats").

RICE: Rest, Ice, Compression, and Elevation. A healing prescription used on some injuries; ice is the most-often-used component, but compression wear (or an ACE bandage), rest, and putting that foot/ankle/knee higher than your heart is never a bad idea.

River Nile: Sweat running between the girls on hot, humid days of summer.

Rulking: More running than walking.

Rumace: Running and grimacing. Often up a hill.

Run for the roses: Marathon in which an athlete attempts to qualify for Boston.

Runiversary: Anniversary of your first run.

Runner's high: Legal in all 50 states and countries worldwide, this is an as-yet-unproven feeling of supreme well-being and elation experienced by some runners after an amazing run. In short: the running equivalent of an orgasm.

S

Sahara: Killer stretches, generally uphill, that have no trees for shade.

Slaying the dragon: Getting out that all-important number two, pre-race, with just minutes before the gun goes off. Often occasion for a little celebration.

Sliming yourself: Condition that occurs when your own **snot rocket** lands on you.

Sloggun: Slippery, soggy runs on snow-covered, icy, melting trails or streets.

Snot rocket: Blowing your nose, sans Kleenex. *Synonyms*: air hanky; farmer blow.

Snot snipered: Unfortunate situation when

you pass another runner right as they are blowing a **snot rocket**.

Split: A delicious concoction made with ice cream, chocolate sauce, and . . . Oh, not *that* kind, sorry. In the running world, a split is the amount of time you take to run a specific segment of a race. Can be mile by mile ("My split for that last mile was blazing fast.") or averaged over the course of a race. For example, if you cross the line of a 10K in 56 minutes flat, you had 9:00 splits, meaning you averaged 9 minutes for each mile.

Spurts: Exertion-induced, unexpected pee leaks.

Step sister: A best running buddy. *Synonym*: sole sister, **BRF**.

Stretching: Something we should all do more of, but that gets cast aside in favor of an extra 5 minutes of running or unloading the dishwasher before the troops awaken.

Strides: An efficient way to develop speed and faster footfalls, strides are usually done at the end of an easy run to remind your legs how to move fast without doing a full hard workout. Involves speeding up for roughly 100 meters (or about 30 seconds), then recovering for about the same amount of time before doing it again.

Swamp ass: Too much sweat between the crack.

Swass: Sweaty Ass.

T

Talking to the cornstalks: Answering nature's call on a rural run. *Synonym*: **Tying your shoe**.

Taper: A beautiful time in a race plan, when you lay off the miles so your muscles can soak up all the hard work you've done and you can head to the starting line rarin' to go. Also a common time to go stir-crazy, especially if you're training for a half or full marathon, but realize it's for the good of the cause. Do *not* run off the crazies.

Tempo: A portion of a run done at 75 to 85 percent of your max effort for a set amount of distance (usually 1 to 4 miles), preceded by a warm-up and followed by a cooldown. Best accompanied by fast-paced tunes or a speedy friend with whom you feel slightly competitive.

Therapy session: A run.

Turnover: How quickly you pick 'em up and lay 'em down ('em = your feet). See also **cadence**.

Tying your shoe: Ducking off for a potty break on a group run.

U

Ultramarathon: Any race longer than 26.2 miles. More often than not, the race is on trails, so runners often hike or power-walk up steep hills to conserve their energy. SBS is alternately intrigued—and horrified—by the idea of running a 50K; Dimity needs to make it through her next half-marathon before she can even think about going farther.

W

Walunning: More walking than running.

Warm-up: The start of most every run, when you run at an ease-into-it pace, hoping your neighbors don't think you *always* run this slowly. It's the time to get your muscles, joints, and (creaky) connective tissues limber and lubed, and to get your head in the game for the upcoming workout.

Wogging: A cross between walking and **jogging** (ick, that word again!).

X

x: A way to abbreviate track workouts. The letter *x* stands for *times*, so 3 x 800 means you run an 800 (twice around the track) three times.

XXX Training: Post-run action in the sack; often brought on by a stronger libido because of revved-up blood flow. *Synonym:* crosstraining.

Z

Zen runner: A runner who won't wave, smile, nod, look, or in any way acknowledge your presence as you pass by. (We generally give them the benefit of the doubt and assume they're in "the zone," otherwise we'd call them something else.)